КИС

Neuropathology

Diagnostic Pathology of Skeletal Muscle and Nerve

Sydney S. Schochet, Jr., M.D.

Department of Pathology, Neurology and Neurosurgery
West Virginia University Medical Center
Morgantown, West Virginia

APPLETON-CENTURY-CROFTS/Norwalk, Connecticut

*This book is dedicated to my colleagues
in neurology, both past and present.*

86 87 88 89 90 / 10 9 8 7 6 5 4 3 2 1

Prentice-Hall of Australia, Pty. Ltd., Sydney
Prentice-Hall Canada, Inc.
Prentice-Hall Hispanoamericana, S. A., Mexico
Prentice-Hall of India Private Limited, New Delhi
Prentice-Hall International (UK) Limited, London
Prentice-Hall of Japan, Inc., Tokyo
Prentice-Hall of Southeast Asia (Pte.) Ltd., Singapore
Whitehall Books Ltd., Wellington, New Zealand
Editora Prentice-Hall do Brasil Ltda., Rio de Janeiro

Library of Congress Cataloging-in-Publication Data

Schochet, Sydney S., 1937–
  Diagnostic pathology of skeletal muscle and nerve.

  Includes index.
  1. Neuromuscular diseases—Diagnosis. 2. History,
Pathological. I. Title. [DNLM: 1. Muscular Diseases
—diagnosis. 2. Muscles—pathology. 3. Peripheral
Nerve Diseases—diagnosis. 4. Peripheral Nerves—
pathology. WE 550 S363d]
RC925.6.S36 1986   616.7'4075   86–3576
ISBN 0–8385–1598–3

PRINTED IN THE UNITED STATES OF AMERICA

Contents

Preface

The objective of this book is to provide a practical guide for individuals who are evaluating morphologic changes in specimens of skeletal muscle and peripheral nerve. It is important to realize that the spectrum of morphologic changes exhibited by these tissues is limited. In many instances, the histopathologic findings merely contribute to the establishment of a definitive diagnosis. It is the author's opinion that appropriate interpretations can be rendered only in the context of the clinical situation. For that reason, brief clinical discussions are included along with the descriptions of the histopathologic features.

The author thanks his many clinical colleagues for making these cases available for study. The author also thanks Ms. Linda Kent Tomago for typing and retyping the manuscript; and Ms. Sally Anderson and Ms. Patricia Turner for preparing the illustrations and Dr. Jeannie Nelson for reviewing the manuscript.

chapter 1

Normal Muscle and General Techniques

Close collaboration between the clinician and the pathologist is essential for the optimal utilization of the muscle biopsy in the diagnosis of neuromuscular and systemic diseases. Muscle biopsy should be undertaken only after the appropriate preliminary data have been acquired. These include a careful history, a thorough physical examination, appropriate electrodiagnostic studies, and appropriate clinical laboratory studies.

Although there are numerous, diverse disorders affecting skeletal muscles, they give rise to relatively few symptoms, principally pain or weakness. The distribution of these complaints and any temporal variations must be documented. In general, difficulty in rising from a chair, running, or climbing are common complaints associated with proximal weakness. Difficulty descending steps, tripping, and clumsiness of the hands are often manifestations of distal weakness. Since many of the neuromuscular diseases and systemic diseases in which muscle biopsies may be employed are hereditary, information regarding other members of the family must be included as an integral part of the historical data. Important signs of neuromuscular disease include manifestations of weakness, muscular wasting, atrophy, fasciculations, pseudohypertrophy, and myotonia. The distribution of the weakness should be documented by recording the strength of individual muscles and muscle groups. This can be accomplished by tabulating the strength with a numerical scale such as the Medical Research Council Scale or more simply, by giving a functional evaluation based on performance of various simple tasks. This approach has been outlined in detail by Brooke.[1] In general, proximal weakness is more often the result of myopathic disorders while distal weakness is more typical of neurogenic processes. Pain or tenderness on palpation is often indicative of inflammatory disorders. Fasciculations should be carefully sought since they are commonly encountered in neurogenic processes. Myotonia, an abnormally slow relaxation of contracted muscles, may be manifested by a "clinging" grip when shaking hands or may be elicited by percussion or having the patient tightly close the eyelids. This phenomenon is an important manifestation of myotonic dystrophy and the other myotonic disorders. Evaluation of the deep tendon reflexes is an important component of the examination for suspected neuromuscular disorders.

The electrodiagnostic studies should include electromyography and nerve conduction studies. The electromyogram (EMG) is an analysis of muscle action potentials and provides valuable indications as to the nature of the muscle disorder, i.e., whether the disorder is neurogenic or myopathic. It is especially valuable in detecting myotonia associated with myotonic dystrophy and the other myotonic disorders. In addition, "electrical myotonia," myotonic discharges detected electrically but not manifested clinically, may be present in various storage disorders. The electromyographic studies aid in determining the distribution of a neuromuscular disorder and facilitating the selection of a muscle that is appropriate for biopsy. The sites actually used for the electromyographic needle studies must be avoided because of resulting inflammation. A suitable biopsy specimen often can be obtained from the corresponding muscle on the opposite side of the body. The nerve conduction studies may include both motor nerve conduction velocities and evaluation of sensory nerve action potentials. The results of these studies are often considerably more significant in evaluating the findings in peripheral nerve biopsy specimens than muscle biopsy specimens. In general, neurogenic atrophy and fiber type grouping (reinnervation) are expected to be associated with axonal degeneration rather than demyelination.

Among the clinical laboratory studies, the creatine phosphokinase (CK) level and the erythrocyte sedimentation rate (ESR) are of special significance in evaluation of neuromuscular diseases. The CK may be markedly elevated in various rapidly evolving myopathies such as Duchenne muscular dystrophy, rhabdomyolysis, and some inflammatory myopathies. Lesser elevations may be seen in other dystrophies, many inflammatory myopathies, and some chronic metabolic myopathies. Mild elevation may even be seen with neurogenic disorders. Elevation of the ESR is expected primarily in the inflammatory myopathies.

The preceding comments are by no means a comprehensive account of the clinical manifestations of neuromuscular disease but provide a brief outline of some of the clinical features and laboratory studies that should be evaluated before the decision is made to perform a muscle biopsy.

PERFORMANCE OF THE MUSCLE BIOPSY

The muscle specimen should be obtained from a moderately involved muscle in severely affected patients or from the most severely involved muscle in early or mildly affected individuals. Sites of recent injections, punctures by EMG needles, and sites of previous surgery should be avoided. The biceps brachii and quadriceps femoris are the preferred muscles when all other considerations are the same. The deltoid muscles should be avoided in adults since they are a repository for a lifetime of injections and are remarkably uninvolved in certain disorders such as facioscapulohumeral dystrophy. The gastrocnemius, despite the ease with which it can be biopsied, should be avoided since the muscle fibers are oriented obliquely and are difficult to section transversely. Furthermore, children with Duchenne muscular dystrophy may become prematurely chair-bound following biopsy of the gastrocnemius. Tendon and fascial insertions should be avoided because of special morphologic features that potentially could be misinterpreted as pathologic alterations. In many instances, the midportion of the muscle, where the motor innervation is located, is the best site. Muscle specimens, obtained from "unusual sites" during surgery for other reasons, often pose special problems in interpretation since the pathologist is generally less familiar with the appearance of normal muscle from these areas. Eye muscles are especially difficult to evaluate.

Generally the biopsy should be done under local anesthesia with the anesthetic agent infiltrated about, but not into, the tissue to be removed. In some young children, it may be necessary to use general anesthesia, however, this should be avoided if possible. When general anesthesia is used, the muscle biopsy is a potentially dangerous procedure since certain neuromuscular diseases potentiate the risk of cardiac arrhythmias and malignant hyperthermia. The specimen must be of sufficient size to permit the appropriate studies to be performed. One or more pieces of tissue, approximately 1 cm in length and about 0.5 cm in diameter are generally sufficient. Many laboratories now do all studies, histologic, morphometric, and histochemical, on frozen tissue. For these procedures, a muscle biopsy clamp is not necessary and in fact, is often wasteful of the tissue. The use of a clamp is most helpful in avoiding excessive contraction artifacts when a portion of the tissue is to be placed directly in formalin or other fixatives.

After excision, the biopsy specimen should be wrapped in gauze moistened with saline. The tissue should then be taken promptly to the histology laboratory for further preparation. Delays should be avoided but they do not necessarily negate the utilization of the specimen for diagnostic purposes. For example, muscle specimens, removed in facilities that are not equipped to perform rapid freezing with liquid nitrogen, can be kept cool (but not frozen!) with ice and transported to a referral laboratory. Satisfactory diagnostic studies can generally be performed if the time from removal to rapid freezing does not exceed a couple hours. Similarly, limited but still informative studies can be performed on muscle specimens obtained from autopsies even when the postmortem interval is several hours in duration.

SPECIMEN PREPARATION

Once in the laboratory, the muscle biopsy specimen should be trimmed to form a small cylinder about 0.5 cm in length and of an equal or lesser diameter. The specimen can be placed directly on a microtome chuck or placed on a small piece of cork (Fig. 1-1). It is essential that the specimen is oriented perpendicularly so that transverse sections can be cut. If there is any doubt regarding orientation, the specimen should be inspected with a dissecting microscope. The muscle is supported by surrounding it with one of the commercial frozen section mounting compounds or thick (about 10 percent) gum tragacanth.

While the muscle specimen is being trimmed and oriented, isopentane (methyl butane), in a wide-mouth cup, should be cooled by immersion in liquid nitrogen. The objective is to very rapidly freeze the muscle in order to avoid artifacts from the formation of ice crystals in the tissue. The very low temperature of liquid nitrogen, about − 160C, is ideal for this purpose. The use of isopentane avoids the formation of an insulating layer of gaseous nitrogen that would retard the freezing process if the muscle were immersed directly in the liquid nitrogen. The isopentane is assumed to be sufficiently cold when small cakes of solid isopentane appear at the bottom and along the sides of the cup. At that time, the muscle specimen and accompanying cork or chuck should be plunged rapidly and without hesitation into the cold isopentane (Fig. 1-2). Any delay in getting the specimen beneath the surface of the cold isopentane will result in the formation of ice crystals since the specimen freezes more slowly in the cold atmosphere above the freezing mixture. Hesitation in immersing the specimen is one of the most common causes of ice crystal artifacts in the sections (Fig. 1-3). The specimen can be left in the cold isopentane for 20 to 30 seconds to become adequately frozen. If the specimen is accidentally distorted by striking the bottom of the container, the specimen can be thawed, reoriented, and rapidly refrozen.

Once frozen, the specimen and underlying cork can be mounted on a microtome chuck with mounting medium, gum tragacanth, or even water prior

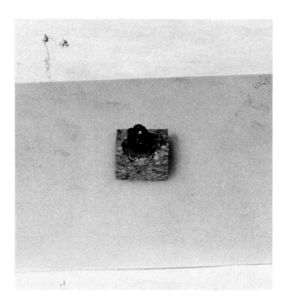

Figure 1-1. The muscle biopsy specimen is mounted on a cork with a commercial frozen section mounting compound or gum tragacanth.

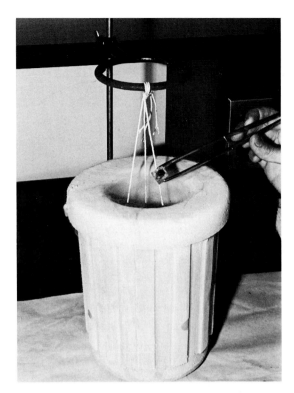

Figure 1-2. The muscle biopsy specimen, mounted on a cork with the frozen section mounting compound, should be plunged rapidly into isopentane that has been cooled with liquid nitrogen. This is the step that must be done very rapidly in order to avoid ice crystal artifacts.

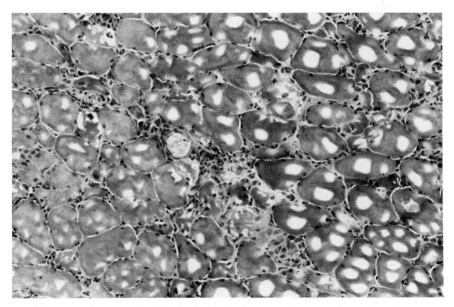

Figure 1-3. Ice crystal artifacts. These holes result from the formation of ice crystals when the tissue has frozen too slowly. H&E, ×175.

to sectioning in a cryostat. Alternatively, the specimen can be stored in a −70 to −85C freezer or shipped on dry ice to another laboratory for sectioning. If the specimen is to be shipped, it should be wrapped in metal foil or enclosed in a thick plastic bag in order to avoid dehydration.

We have found a cryostat setting of −20C to be satisfactory for most specimens. Those containing unusually large amounts of adipose tissue may cut better at a lower temperature but often yield poor quality sections despite all efforts. It is important to use a well-sharpened microtome knife and use of an antiroll device is a great help (Fig. 1–4). Satisfactory sections generally can be cut using a setting of 10 to 12 μm. The microscope slides that are used to pick up the sections should be thoroughly cleaned to avoid artifacts from poor adherence. Some laboratories prefer to use coverslips for the sections but these are more difficult to handle and cannot be labeled ahead of time. They do permit the use of smaller quantities of staining solutions. The slides with the attached sections may be kept overnight before carrying out the staining reactions without any serious loss of reactivity. For longer delays, e.g., over the weekend, the sections may be stored in the −70 to −85C freezer. After all of the frozen sections have been cut, the specimen with attached cork can be placed in a small plastic container for indefinite storage in the freezer. Alter-

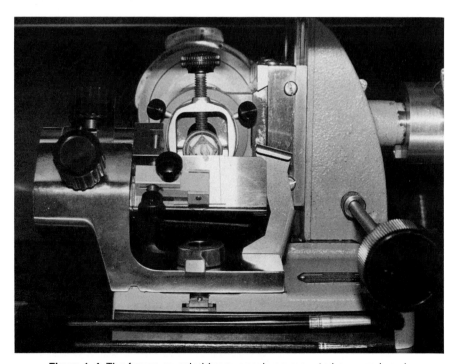

Figure 1-4. The frozen muscle biopsy specimen mounted on a cork and attached to the chuck of the microtome. We find a temperature of about −20C to be suitable for sectioning most specimens.

natively, the remainder of the specimen can be placed in formalin and fixed for subsequent paraffin-embedded sections. In actual practice, we often use two specimens, one of which we keep frozen and the other we submit for formalin fixation and paraffin-embedded sections. The tissue that is stored frozen can be resectioned if additional histochemical reactions are needed or can be used for subsequent biochemical studies. It is generally desirable to have a portion of the tissue embedded in paraffin since these sections are occasionally superior to frozen sections for evaluating vasculitis. Also, the paraffin blocks provide a permanent repository for a portion of the specimen.

Electron microscopy is a valuable adjunct procedure in the evaluation of a small number of carefully selected patients. We usually fix a small portion of the tissue in cacodylate-buffered glutaraldehyde and save it for subsequent epoxy embedment. We select a small fascicle of the biopsy specimen from beneath the surface, away from the traumatic artifacts produced by the surgical procedure. The specimen must be gently stretched and supported while undergoing fixation. We accomplish this by letting the fascicle of muscle adhere to an applicator stick or to the frosted end of a microscope slide before immersion in the glutaraldehyde. Only after the specimen is at least partially fixed do we cut the tissue into small cubes measuring 1 mm or less. Subsequently, the tissue is postfixed in cacodylate-buffered osmium tetroxide solution. We routinely block stain the tissue with magnesium uranyl acetate solution in order to enhance the contrast for electron microscopy. Occasionally, additional blocks are processed without the use of the block stain since this solution tends to leach glycogen out of the specimen. After dehydration in alcohols, the specimen is placed in propylene oxide and embedded in an epoxy resin. We often prepare "thick sections" that are stained with toluidine blue for light microscopy even when electron microscopy is not contemplated. The actual electron microscopy is never undertaken until all of the frozen sections, paraffin-embedded sections, and epoxy sections have been completely studied by light microscopy.

STAINS EMPLOYED ON FROZEN SECTIONS

Since most of the diagnostic interpretations are based on study of the frozen sections, we will briefly discuss the battery of stains that we employ routinely and indicate the rationale for the use of each.

Hematoxylin and Eosin (H&E)

This is a rapid, reliable staining procedure which provides a good overview of any pathologic changes that may be present. When the sections are not cut too thinly, the type I myofibers stain slightly darker than the type II myofibers (Fig. 1–5). Thus this stain even provides some preliminary information regarding the presence and distribution of the two major fiber types. It is the best of the techniques employed on frozen sections for the detection of vasculitis and inflammatory cell infiltrates.

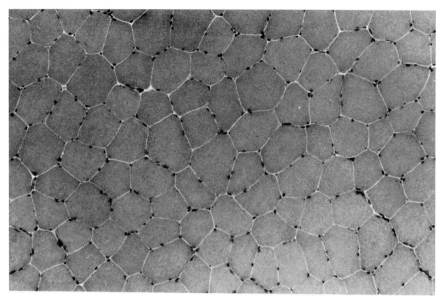

Figure 1-5. Frozen section stained with H&E. This is a good survey stain. Note the polygonal shape of the myofibers and peripheral location of the myofiber nuclei. The type I myofibers stain slightly darker and are slightly smaller than the type II myofibers. ×175.

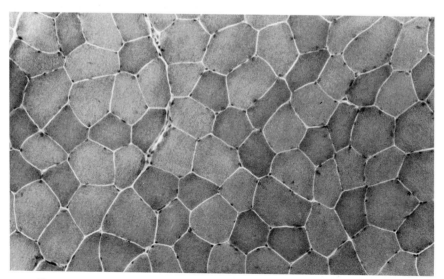

Figure 1-6. Frozen section stained with the modified trichrome stain. A good survey stain. The type I myofibers stain a darker green than the type II myofibers. ×180.

Modified Gomori Trichrome

This is another good survey stain for overall evaluation of pathologic changes. We employ the "superchrome" modification of Engel and Cunningham.[2] When applied to unfixed, frozen sections, the resulting colors are quite different from those seen with formalin-fixed tissue. The muscle fibers stain bluish–green, and in many cases, the type I myofibers stain somewhat more darkly than the type II myofibers (Fig. 1–6). Connective tissue is also stained green but tends to be much lighter and of a different hue than the muscle. Certain pathologic processes are vividly portrayed by this technique. Abnormal focal accumulations of mitochondria stain red and the fibers so affected are designated as "ragged-red" fibers. Many abnormal inclusions such as nemaline rods, cytoplasmic bodies, phospholipid deposits in "rimmed vacuoles," and other deposits in autophagic vacuoles are stained various shades of red to purple. Target fibers, an alteration characteristically associated with denervating disorders, are often visualized readily with the trichrome stain. In addition, myelinated nerve fibers within the biopsy specimen are seen distinctly. The myelin stains red and appears somewhat vacuolated while the contained axons are darker and blue–green in color.

Periodic Acid Schiff (PAS)

This stain results from the reaction of periodic acid on vicinal hydroxy-, or vicinal hydroxy- and amino-groups to produce colored complexes with the Schiff reagent. The type II myofibers, especially the type IIB myofibers, stain somewhat more darkly than the type I myofibers. This, however, is not a reliable stain for distinguishing the two major fiber types. Most of the staining in muscle fibers is due to the presence of normal or abnormal deposits of glycogen. In order to identify glycogen with greater certainty, successive sections can be stained with and without prior digestion with amylase or diastase (the diastase in saliva is often sufficient). Necrotic fibers are often unstained. The PAS reaction also stains the basement membrane and plasmalemma about myofibers. Thus this technique serves to accentuate the shape of the myofibers and facilitates the recognition of abnormally small or irregular fibers. Sections stained by the PAS reaction are quite suitable for the detection of target fibers and ring fibers. Fibers showing the latter alteration can be further demonstrated by examining the sections with polarized light.

Nicotinamide Adenine Dinucleotide–Tetrazolium Reductase (NADH-TR)

This stain is primarily a histochemical reaction for oxidative enzyme activity. For this reason, the type I myofibers are stained darker than the type II myofibers and the procedure has at least limited application for distinguishing the major fiber types (Fig. 1–7). The NADH–TR reaction stains atrophic, denervated fibers darkly regardless of their type. This reaction, in conjunction with the nonspecific esterase reaction, is helpful in detecting small numbers of atrophic denervated myofibers. It is the best technique available for the detec-

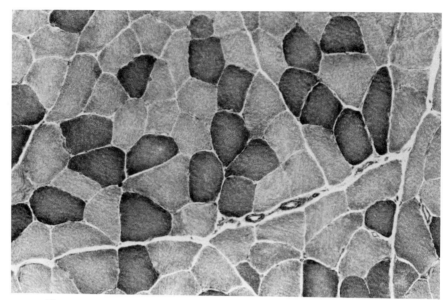

Figure 1-7. Frozen section stained with the NADH–TR reaction. The type I myofibers stain a darker blue but this is not a reliable stain for fiber typing. ×175.

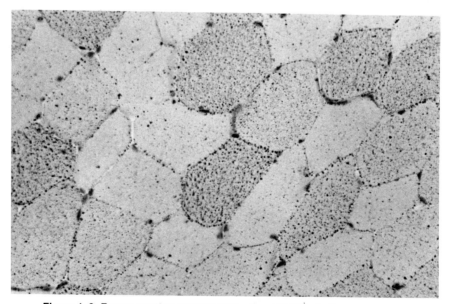

Figure 1-8. Frozen section stained with oil red O. This is the most commonly employed stain for evaluation of lipid content. The type I myofibers contain more lipid droplets. Clean preparations are difficult to obtain. ×440.

tion of target fibers. This alteration occurs almost exclusively in type I my-ofibers. The central portion of the target fiber is unstained. This area is surrounded by a zone of enhanced staining while the periphery of the myofiber is stained normally. Targetoid fibers, cores, and so-called "moth-eaten" fibers are also clearly demonstrated. Mitochondrial aggregates are stained darkly. Components of this stain also react with the sarcoplasmic reticulum and its derivatives. For example, tubular aggregates, as seen in the periodic paralyses, are stained.

Succinic Dehydrogenase (SDH)

This is another histochemical reaction for oxidative enzyme activity but is more specific for mitochondria. This reaction is generally used to determine whether dark-staining deposits detected with the NADH–TR reaction are due to mi-tochondria or some other tissue component, e.g., tubular aggregates stain darkly with the NADH–TR reaction but remain unstained with the SDH procedure.

Oil Red O

This stain is commonly employed for the detection of neutral lipid droplets. These appear as punctate dots and are more abundant in the type I than the type II myofibers (Fig. 1–8). The staining depends on the selective extraction of the dye by the lipid droplets in which it is more soluble than water. Un-fortunately, sections stained by this technique are often difficult to interpret because of spurious deposition of the dye. An excessive content of stainable neutral lipid is seen in certain of the lipid storage and mitochondrial myopa-thies. The myelin sheaths of intramuscular nerve twigs are also stained in these preparations.

Osmium Tetroxide–Paraphenylenediamine (Os–PPD)

This stain was developed in our laboratory[3] from techniques previously em-ployed for the staining of epoxy sections. This methodology was in turn based on procedures devised many years ago for staining myelin in sections of central nervous system tissue. In many cases, this stain provides preparations that are less contaminated by spurious deposits of dye than the oil red O-stained sec-tions. Deposits of mitochondria, droplets of neutral lipid, and possibly other lipids are stained (Fig. 1–9). This technique also stains the myelin sheaths of nerve within muscle biopsy specimens.

Acid Phosphatase

This reaction is used as a marker for increased lysosomal activity. Deposits of the reaction product are seen in necrotic and degenerating myofibers in diverse conditions such as rhabdomyolysis, certain inflammatory myopathies, and cer-tain dystrophies, especially Duchenne muscular dystrophy. Markedly increased acid phosphatase activity is seen in lysosomal storage diseases such as type II glycogenosis. In the adult form of the latter disease, small punctate foci of acid phosphatase activity are encountered even in myofibers that do not contain

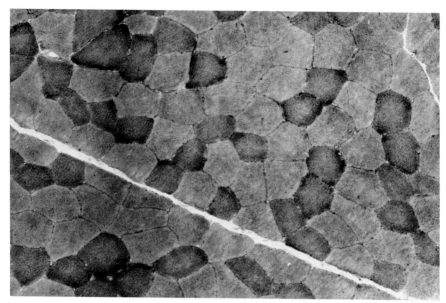

Figure 1-9. Frozen section stained with Os-PPD. This stain will often provide cleaner preparations, however, the staining is not restricted to triglycerides. × 175.

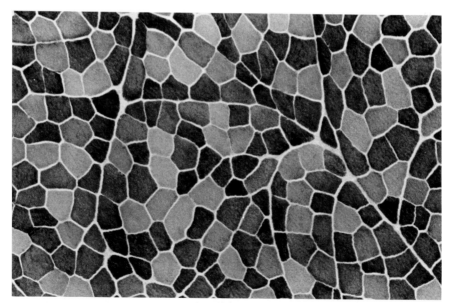

Figure 1-10. Frozen section stained with the myophosphorylase reaction. Note the type II fibers are stained darker than the type I myofibers. In cases of myophosphorylase deficiency, the slide will appear nearly unstained even without the use of the microscope (see Fig. 6-27 for example of McArdle's disease). × 175.

conspicuous storage vacuoles. The ceroid deposits associated with the ceroid-lipofuscinoses and lipofuscin deposits associated with myotonic dystrophy and advanced aging show increased acid phosphatase activity. Little or no acid phosphatase activity is seen in normal muscle.

Alkaline Phosphatase
This reaction is used mainly for the demonstration of abnormally reactive blood vessels and connective tissue in certain of the inflammatory myopathies. This technique also stains regenerating myofibers regardless of their cause. Under some circumstances, denervated muscle will show some increased reactivity. Little or no alkaline phosphatase activity is seen in specimens of normal skeletal muscle.

Myophosphorylase
This enzymatic reaction is based on reversal of the normal phosphorylase reaction in skeletal muscle and detects, with the use of iodine, the presence of glycogen. The absence of this enzymatic activity throughout the muscle biopsy specimen is virtually diagnostic of myophosphorylase deficiency, regardless of whether it is due to absence or inactivity of the enzyme.[4] This staining reaction will stain normal type II myofibers more darkly than type I myofibers (Fig. 1–10). Enzyme deficiency is manifested by virtually no staining. Preparations suspected of showing enzyme deficiency must be carefully monitored with control material. This is most readily done by mounting sections from the patient and a normal control subject on the same slide before performing the staining process. Necrotic myofibers, regardless of their cause, will show absence of the enzyme reaction. Conversely, regenerating myofibers in specimens from patients with myophosphorylase deficiency may show staining due to the presence of certain myophosphorylase isoenzymes. This stain will also vividly demonstrate target fibers in some cases of denervating disease.

Nonspecific Esterase
The precise histochemical basis for the staining of muscle fibers with this procedure is unknown. We have modified the standard methodology by using crude basic fuchsin rather than the more highly purified pararosanaline. The standard procedure results in very pale staining of normal myofibers. Our modified procedure results in overall more intense staining with the type I myofibers staining darker than the type II myofibers (Fig. 1–11). Furthermore, subtypes of the type I myofibers are recognizable by variation in the degree of staining. Myoneural junctions are prominently stained. In addition, inflammatory cells show intense staining. The major diagnostic application of this technique is to facilitate the detection of small numbers of atrophic denervated myofibers. These fibers are stained darkly, as with the NADH–TR reaction, regardless of their fiber type. The intense brown color is easily seen in contrast to the yellow and light brown colors of the normally innervated myofibers.

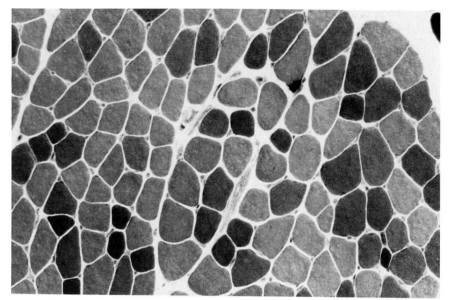

Figure 1-11. Frozen section stained with the nonspecific esterase reaction. The type I myofibers stain brown while the type II myofibers stain dark yellow. ×175.

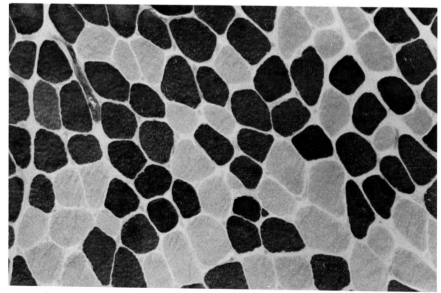

Figure 1-12. Frozen section stained with myofibrillar ATPase at pH 9.4. The type II myofibers stain dark brown while the type I myofibers are lighter. This is the standard fiber typing reaction to which all other procedures are compared. ×220.

Myofibrillar Adenosine Triphosphatase (ATPase)

This reaction is the standard procedure for classifying myofibers into the various fiber types.[5] The basic reaction is carried out under very alkaline conditions, pH 9.4 or higher. Under these conditions, the type II myofibers stain dark brown while the type I myofibers stain light brown (Fig. 1–12). The basic procedure is often supplemented by preincubation of the sections in acidic buffers. Preincubation in a buffer at pH 4.3 results in a reversal of the previous staining reaction, i.e., the type I fibers are stained dark brown and the type II myofibers are very palely stained if at all. A few type II fibers will be faintly stained; these are designated as type IIC or undifferentiated fibers. Classification can be further refined by staining additional sections that have been preincubated in a buffer at pH 4.6. Under these conditions, the type IIA fibers are lightly stained while the type IIB and the type I myofibers are darkly stained. We routinely perform the basic reaction at pH 9.4 to 10.4 and the supplemental reaction with sections preincubated at pH 4.3. We do not routinely employ the intermediate pH 4.6 incubation since most diagnostic studies are adequately conducted with a two-fiber classification, i.e., type I or type II, without resorting to further subclassification. Although these stains are invaluable for evaluating the relative number, size, and distribution of the fiber types, relatively few of the other pathologic alterations can be seen. Target fibers are a noteworthy exception and appear as type I myofibers with an unstained central zone.

Congo Red or Crystal Violet

These stains are occasionally employed for the detection of amyloid. The Congo Red reaction is more suitable when performed on paraffin-embedded sections.

Myoadenylate Deaminase (MAD)

This histochemical reaction was introduced relatively recently[6] to detect deficiency of this enzyme which is part of the purine nucleotide cycle. Although this reaction is not yet a part of the standard histochemical battery in many laboratories including our own, it is undergoing extensive evaluation. Deficiency of MAD has been reported in certain patients with weakness and cramps, in occasional normal individuals, and in a wide variety of unrelated neuromuscular conditions.

STAINS EMPLOYED ON PARAFFIN-EMBEDDED SECTIONS

Although frozen sections are generally the most satisfactory technique for diagnostic studies on skeletal muscle, paraffin-embedded sections are still useful for certain purposes. A portion of the biopsy specimen, often the remainder of the tissue previously used for the frozen sections can be fixed in formalin and processed for paraffin-embedded sections. This is done to provide "archival" storage of the muscle biopsy specimens along with other surgical specimens without the problems associated with prolonged storage of tissue in freezers. Furthermore, inflammatory cell infiltrates and amyloid deposits are often easier to detect in the paraffin-embedded sections than in the frozen sections. Occasionally, a muscle biopsy will be handled improperly and placed directly in formalin. Under these circumstances, one must attempt to make maximal utilization of the paraffin-embedded sections since the frozen sections and the stains usually performed on them are no longer possible. Finally, multiple tissue samples may be taken from various sites when performing an autopsy. Some of the specimens can be processed as frozen sections, but it is often impractical to handle all of the specimens in this fashion. The remainder are usually processed as paraffin-embedded tissue. Especially with tissue from autopsies, fixation in Heidenhain's SUSA solution may yield sections that are superior to formalin fixation if the specimens are sufficiently small and fixed properly. Careful attention must be given to the length of fixation to avoid overfixation and the tissue must receive proper treatment to avoid contamination from the mercury. The SUSA fixative is highly toxic and must be handled carefully and disposed of properly. An additional advantage of the paraffin-embedded sections is the ability to prepare both longitudinal and cross-sections. We have found a battery of four stains—H&E, trichrome, PAS, and phosphotungstic acid hematoxylin (PTAH)—that routinely yield the maximal information. Other stains such as Congo Red are performed only when indicated by clinical data or other morphologic findings.

NORMAL SKELETAL MUSCLE

The muscle fibers that constitute an anatomically defined muscle are bound together by a connective tissue sheath, the epimysium. This is in continuity with the connective tissue of the periosteum, tendons, and aponeuroses at the origins and insertions of the muscle. The perimysium consists of connective tissue septa that divide the muscle into fascicles. Individual muscle fibers or myofibers are separated from one another by a small amount of connective tissue that constitutes the endomysium. The myofibers are long multinucleated cells that extend without interruption from the origin to the insertion of a muscle or muscle fascicle. Since the fascicles in most muscles are arranged in a pennate fashion, most myofibers do not exceed 10 cm in length. The average diameter of the myofibers varies with age, sex, and physical development. Infants and children obviously have smaller myofibers than adults. In infancy, the myofibers measure only about 15 μm in diameter. This gradually increases throughout childhood. Adult dimensions are generally not achieved until the individual is 10 to 20 years of age. For this reason, it is necessary to measure the myofibers and determine their average size when evaluating specimens from children. A very useful graph of the mean myofiber diameters at various ages as determined from frozen sections can be found in the monograph by Dubowitz and Brooke.[7] Myofibers, especially type II myofibers, from women are generally smaller than from men of comparable age. In men the type I myofibers generally measure 60 to 65 μm in diameter while the type II myofibers measure 60 to 70 μm in diameter. In women, fibers of both types are more nearly the same size and average 40 to 50 μm in diameter. The type II myofibers are especially sensitive to physical activity and tend to become enlarged ("work hypertrophy") in individuals of either sex who do strenuous labor or engage in vigorous exercise. There is also variation from muscle to muscle within a given individual. The myofibers in the large antigravity muscles tend to be larger than in the small distal muscles. Because of this regional variation, it is easier to interpret specimens from the "standard" biopsy sites than from less frequently sampled sites. This is one of the major problems in evaluating muscle specimens from nonconventional sites obtained during the course of a surgical procedure. The spectrum of fiber sizes in both normal muscle and pathologic conditions can be vividly portrayed by the use of histograms.[7]

ULTRASTRUCTURE OF SKELETAL MUSCLE

The surface of the myofiber itself, the plasmalemma, contains multiple small invaginations, the caveolae, and often appears undercoated by a discontinuous band of finely granular osmiophilic material (Fig. 1–13). The term sarcolemma, often used as a synonym for the plasmalemma, was also used previously by light microscopists, in which case it also included the overlying basement membrane and adherent collagenous fibers from the endomysium. The latter structures persist even when the myofiber degenerates.

Myofiber nuclei are normally found immediately beneath the plasmalemma. Their location is more readily evaluated in transverse sections than in longitudinal sections where superimposition of myofibers can lead to the spurious appearance of an internal location. Normally no more than about 3 percent of the myofibers should contain internal nuclei. These are often designated as "central nuclei" but only in rare instances do the nuclei even approach a truly central location. When abundant, internal nuclei are indicative of disease; chronic denervation, acquired myopathies, certain hereditary myopathies, and commonly myotonic dystrophy. Internal nuclei may be seen normally adjacent to tendinous and fascial insertions. These areas should be avoided when the biopsy is being performed. The myofiber nuclei have dispersed chromatin and contain one or two nucleoli. Some of the nuclei seen at the surface of a myofiber belong to the satellite cells. These are small, fusiform cells located between the basement membrane and the plasmalemma. They have relatively large nuclei with scanty cytoplasm containing ribosomes and mitochondria but no myofibrils. Normally they account for over 10 percent of the surface nuclei seen in children but only 2 to 5 percent of the peripheral nuclei in adults. They are most numerous in diseased muscle and participate in the regeneration of previously necrotic myofibers.

The contractile elements, the myofilaments are aggregated into myofibrils.

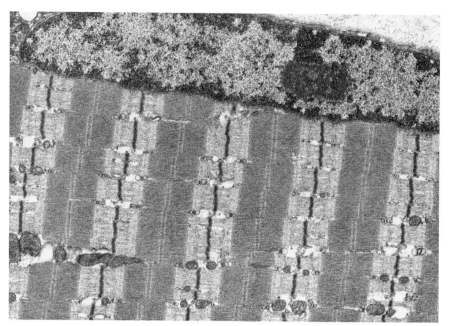

Figure 1-13. Electron micrograph showing normal skeletal muscle in longitudinal section. The surface of the myofiber is covered by a prominent basement membrane. The nucleus is typically elongated and occupies a subsarcolemmal location. The periodically striated myofibrils are composed of myofilaments. × 14,000.

These are periodically banded bundles that are 0.5 to 1.0 μm in diameter and extend the length of the myofiber. Precise alignment of the bands in adjacent myofibrils imparts the characteristic cross striated appearance to the myofiber. By light microscopy, especially with polarized light, the myofiber appears to consist of alternating light and dark bands, i.e., the anisotropic A bands and the isotropic I bands. The myofibrils are divided into repeating linear subunits, the sarcomeres. The sarcomeres vary in length depending upon the degree of muscle contraction. The central portion of the sarcomere contains the A band. It is occupied by parallel thick filaments with thin filaments interdigitating at both ends (Fig. 1–14). The thick filaments are composed predominantly of myosin. The thick myosin filaments measure approximately 1.5 μm in length and 16 nm in diameter. The myosin filaments have a regular hexagonal arrangement that is evident when the myofibril is viewed in cross-section. In the middle of the A band is an osmiophilic area that is termed the M band. In this area, the myosin chains reverse polarity and the thick filaments are interconnected by special cross-bridges. Surrounding the M band is a paler zone of variable width known as the H band. In this portion of the A band there are no interdigitating thin filaments. The I bands contain thin filaments and vary in length depending upon the degree of muscle contraction. The thin filaments

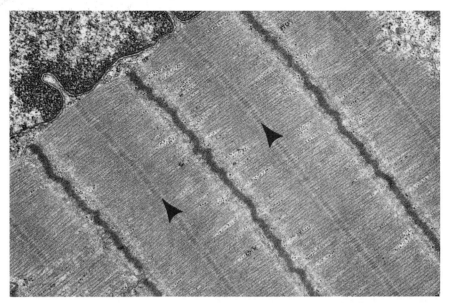

Figure 1-14. Higher-magnification electron micrograph showing the A and I bands. Note the M band *(arrow)* in the middle of the A band. The dark Z-discs divide the myofibril into sarcomeres. ×28,000.

measure approximately 7 nm in diameter and are composed predominantly of actin, troponin, and tropomyosin. When viewed in cross-section, they appear less regularly arranged than the thick filaments. The electron-dense Z-discs have a distinctive woven or quadratic appearance (Fig. 1-15). The detailed ultrastructure and chemical composition of the Z-disc have been the subject of extensive investigations and are still incompletely established. The thin filaments from successive sarcomeres are in some way interconnected and coated with additional proteins which impart the characteristic osmiophilia to the Z-disc.

Each myofibril is accompanied by two complex membranous systems, the sarcoplasmic reticulum and the transverse tubular system. The membranous cisterns of the sarcoplasmic reticulum form a fenestrated network about the exterior of each myofibril. Most of the resulting tubules are oriented parallel to the long axis of the myofibril. The sarcoplasmic reticulum is somewhat more abundant in type II myofibers than in type I myofibers. The transverse tubular system arises from invaginations of the plasmalemma and is in continuity with the extracellular space. The tubules extend inward, perpendicular to the long axis of the myofiber, and encircle the myofibrils. The triads are specialized structures that arise where the transverse tubules periodically intersect the sarcoplasmic reticulum. In human skeletal muscle, each sarcomere is generally accompanied by two triads that tend to overlie the junctions between the A and I bands. Each triad consists of two lateral sacs or terminal cisterns derived

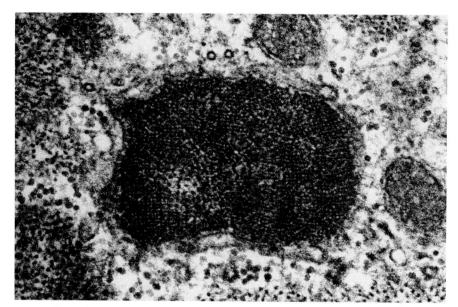

Figure 1-15. High-magnification electron micrograph of skeletal muscle in cross-section. Note the quadratic array of the Z-disc components. ×140,000.

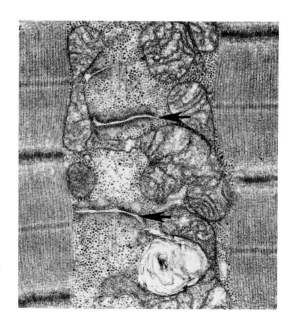

Figure 1-16. High-magnification electron micrograph showing triads *(arrows).* The central T-tubule is flanked on both sides by terminal cisterns of the sarcoplasmic reticulum. ×28,000.

from the sarcoplasmic reticulum flanking a central T-tubule derived from the transverse tubular system (Fig. 1-16). The lateral sacs or terminal cisterns are filled with an amorphous osmiophilic material and appear more electron dense than the T-tubule or the remainder of the sarcoplasmic reticulum. The terminal cisterns have a scalloped margin and are separated from the T-tubule by a narrow gap in which there are small osmiophilic densities referred to as "feet." Thus the two membranous systems are closely apposed but not in continuity.

Myofibers contain abundant mitochondria. These are normally most numerous just beneath the plasmalemma and at the poles of the myofiber nuclei. They are also found in parallel rows between the myofibrils. The mitochondria within the intermyofibrillar spaces tend to overlie the junctions between the A and I bands. Most contain typical transverse cristae although other, more complex, configurations may be encountered. Many of the mitochondria have small dense granules within their matrix compartments. The granules are thought to contain calcium. Mitochondria are somewhat more numerous in type I myofibers than in type II myofibers. Lipid droplets are often found in close relation to mitochondria especially within type I myofibers. The lipid droplets consist predominantly of triglycerides and appear as empty or faintly osmiophilic, homogenous vacuoles. Glycogen deposits are generally most abundant just beneath the plasmalemma, about the poles of the myofiber nuclei, and within the intermyofibrillar spaces. Additional glycogen granules may be interspersed among the myofilaments. The glycogen occurs in the form of small individual granules, so-called beta particles. The myofibers also contain free ribosomes but these are difficult to recognize especially when glycogen granules are abundant. Cisterns of rough endoplasmic reticulum are rarely prominent. A few short cisterns, studded with ribosomes, may be seen adjacent to the myofiber nuclei. Lysosomes, residual bodies, and lipofuscin are generally inconspicuous in normal muscle.

INTRAMUSCULAR BLOOD VESSELS

In addition to the muscle fibers themselves, there are additional structures within the biopsy specimens that must be recognized and evaluated. Muscle contains abundant blood vessels. The larger vessels are readily seen in both frozen and paraffin-embedded sections and are well stained with the H&E and trichrome stains. The larger vessels are also prominently stained by the ATPase techniques on the frozen sections. By contrast, it is very difficult to examine capillaries in the frozen sections. They are recognized mainly by the presence of the endothelial nuclei since the lumens are often not apparent. Type I myofibers are accompanied by more numerous capillaries than type II myofibers. Detailed evaluation of the number and morphology of the capillaries must be performed by light microscopy of epoxy-embedded "thick" sections or by electron microscopy. Even then recognition of pathologic alterations is often difficult since there is marked variation in size, shape, lumenal area, endothelial thickness, and basement membrane thickness.[8,9] Normal capillaries are lined by a single layer of relatively thin endothelial cells that are joined to one another by conspicuous junctional complexes. Numerous pinocytotic vesicles are found on the lumenal and basal surfaces and to a lesser extent, throughout their cytoplasm. In addition to the usual complement of mitochrondia, cisterns of endoplasmic reticulum and intracytoplasmic filaments, occasional Weibel–Palade bodies may be encountered. These distinctive cytosomes have a characteristic tubular internal structure and are a good "marker" for the identification of endothelial cells. The thickness of the basement membrane increases with age, especially in individuals who are over the age of 40, and in various diseases. The degree of thickening is significantly greater in diabetic than nondiabetic individuals.[10] Unfortunately, these measurements are not useful as diagnostic criterion because of the marked individual variation.

INTRAMUSCULAR NERVES AND NEUROMUSCULAR JUNCTIONS

Intramuscular nerve twigs are commonly encountered in the perimysial connective tissue. These are stained by many of the stains used on the frozen and paraffin-embedded sections but are especially well visualized with the modified trichrome and the lipid stains used on the frozen sections. When the muscle biopsy specimens are obtained from near the "motor point," i.e., the site of innervation, smaller terminal ramifications can be seen in the endomysial connective tissue. These lead to the neuromuscular junctions (Figs. 1–17 and 1–18). These structures are readily seen in frozen sections stained with the nonspecific esterase reaction but can be evaluated in detail only by electron microscopy. The nerve twig loses its myelin sheath and branches to a varying degree as it approaches the neuromuscular junction. The distal unmyelinated axon and its terminal expansion are covered by Schwann cell cytoplasm. The terminal ramifications, containing numerous mitochondria and synaptic vesicles, are separated from the muscle fiber by the primary and secondary synaptic clefts (Fig. 1–19). The accumulation of sarcoplasm at the neuromuscular junction results in an elevation called "Doyere's eminence." A thick layer of basement membrane material separates the axon terminal from the synaptic region, the so-called "sole plate" of the myofiber. Additional basement material extends into and fills the invaginations of the secondary synaptic clefts. The sarcoplasm beneath the neuromuscular junctions contains abundant glycogen, mitochondria, and cisterns of endoplasmic reticulum. There are marked variations in the ultrastructural morphology of the neuromuscular junctions. Any alterations should be interpreted with caution and preferably from quantitative data.[11]

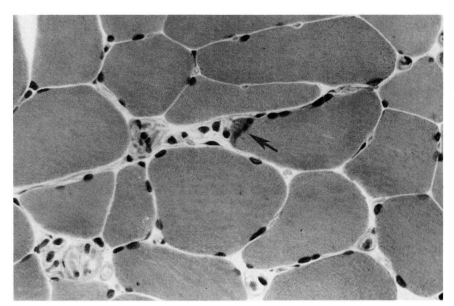

Figure 1-17. Frozen section stained with H&E. Note the neuromuscular junction *(arrow).* ×440.

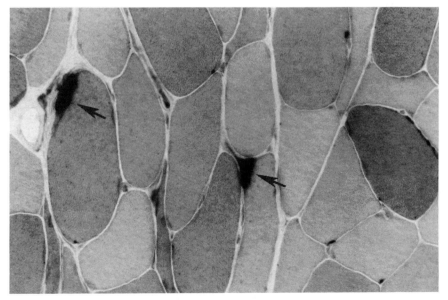

Figure 1-18. Frozen section stained with nonspecific esterase. The neuromuscular junctions *(arrows)* are stained intensely. ×440.

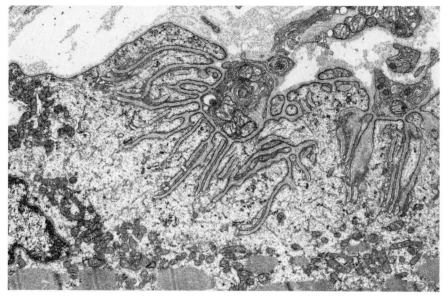

Figure 1-19. Electron micrograph showing a neuromuscular junction. Note the primary synaptic cleft and the numerous "gutters" that comprise the secondary synaptic clefts. ×14,000.

MUSCLE SPINDLES

Another structure that must be recognized and interpreted correctly is the muscle spindle (Figs. 1–20 and 1–21). These fusiform structures provide the central nervous system with information regarding the degree and rate of stretch applied to a skeletal muscle. The spindles consist of a group of specialized muscle fibers that are surrounded in part, by a connective tissue capsule. The spindles usually contain 4 to 16 intrafusal muscle fibers. These are of two types, the nuclear bag fibers and the nuclear chain fibers. The nuclear bag fibers project beyond the capsule at the poles of the spindles. In their midportions, the nuclear bag fibers are expanded and contain collections of many vesicular nuclei. The contractile elements are confined to a thin peripheral band. The nuclear chain fibers arise and insert within the capsule of the spindle. In their midportions, the nuclear chain fibers contain single rows of central nuclei surrounded by abundant contractile components. The capsules are prominent and are composed of concentric lamellae of connective tissue. Gelatinous material may be seen between the capsule and the intrafusal fibers. Nerve twigs and vessels may be seen entering the capsules. The spindles are readily seen in both frozen and paraffin-embedded sections, however, their appearance varies considerably depending on the portion of the spindle included in the section. On occasions, they have been misinterpreted as pathologic changes, either parasites or abnormal myofibers. They will often persist long after the other com-

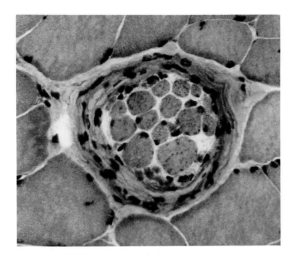

Figure 1-20. Frozen section showing a muscle spindle. The appearance varies somewhat depending on the level of the section. H&E, ×510.

ponents of muscle have undergone atrophy and replacement by fibroadipose tissue. Thus they are an important morphologic feature for establishing that a specimen of fibroadipose tissue had at one time been skeletal muscle. At the present time, few if any diseases can be diagnosed from the appearance of the spindles. An increase in the number of intrafusal fibers has been documented in myotonic dystrophy.[12] However, the other morphologic features are more readily demonstrated in extrafusal myofibers.

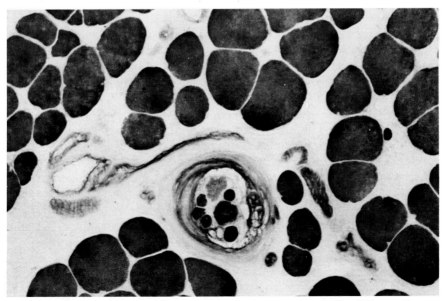

Figure 1-21. Frozen section showing another muscle spindle. ATPase, pH 9.4, ×220.

MUSCLE FIBER TYPING

It has long been recognized that muscle fibers vary in their rate of contraction and their use of substrates for energy production. In many animals, there are whole muscles that are composed almost entirely of fibers of a single type. Commonly cited examples are the pectoral muscles of the chicken, composed almost exclusively of type II myofibers, and the soleus muscle of the rat which is composed predominantly of type I myofibers. The predominance of a single myofiber type imparts the characteristic color and physiologic properties, i.e., "fast-twitch" or "slow-twitch," to the entire muscle. By contrast, human skeletal muscles, at least those that are commonly biopsied, are composed of a mosaic of various types. An important part of the diagnostic evaluation of a muscle biopsy specimen is the determination of the relative number, size, and distribution of these fiber types. One of the major objectives of the earlier histochemical studies on frozen sections was the development of reliable techniques for the typing of muscle fibers. At the present time, the myofibrillar ATPase reaction is the standard technique for muscle fiber typing. As previously outlined, other stains will to some extent distinguish the various fiber types but are not as reliable for routine use. The regular ATPase reaction under alkaline conditions (pH 9.4 to 10.4) clearly delineates two types of myofibers in normal muscle and in most pathologic conditions. The type I myofibers can be subtyped by the use of the nonspecific esterase technique.[13] However, for most diagnostic applications, a two-fiber classification based on the routine ATPase reaction and the ATPase reaction after preincubation at pH 4.3 will suffice.[14] The staining characteristics, some of the ultrastructural features, and the approximate physiologic equivalents are outlined in Table 1–1.

TABLE 1–1. COMPARISON OF TYPE I AND TYPE II MYOFIBERS

	Type I	Type II
Regular ATPase, pH 9.4	Light	Dark
ATPase, preincubated at pH 4.3	Dark	Light
NADH–TR	Dark	Light
PAS	Light	Dark (esp. IIA)
Phosphorylase	Light	Dark
Nonspecific esterase	Dark	Light
H&E	Darker	Lighter
Trichrome	Darker	Lighter
Mitochondria	Abundant	Sparse
Lipid droplets	Abundant	Sparse
Z-disc	Broader	Narrower
M Band	Broader	Narrower
Sarcoplasmic reticulum	Sparse	Abundant
Color	Red	White
Speed of contraction	Slow twitch	Fast twitch

References

1. Brooke MH: A Clinician's View of Neuromuscular Diseases. Baltimore, Williams & Wilkins, 1977, pp 1-33.
2. Engel WK, Cunningham G: Rapid examination of muscle tissue. An improved trichrome method for fresh-frozen biopsy sections. Neurology 13:919-923, 1963.
3. Anderson SC, Schochet SS Jr: Osmium tetroxide-p-phenylenediamine stain for lipid in skeletal muscle. Arch Neurol 39:383, 1982.
4. Feit H, Brooke MH: Myophosphorylase deficiency: Two different molecular etiologies. Neurology 26:963-967, 1976.
5. Brooke MH, Kaiser KK: Muscle fiber types: How many and what kind. Arch Neurol 23:369-379, 1970.
6. Fishbein WN, Griffin JL, Armbrustmacher VW: Stain for skeletal muscle adenylate deaminase. An effective tetrazolium stain for frozen biopsy specimens. Arch Pathol Lab Med 104:462-466, 1980.
7. Dubowitz V, Brooke MH: Muscle Biopsy: A Modern Approach. London, Saunders, 1973.
8. Jerusalem F, Engel AG, Gomez MR: Duchenne dystrophy: I. Morphometric study of the muscle microvasculature. Brain 97:115-122, 1974.
9. Jerusalem F, Rakusa M, Engel AG, MacDonald RD: Morphometric analysis of skeletal muscle capillary ultrastructure in inflammatory myopathies. J Neurol Sci 23:391-402, 1974.
10. Sosenko JM, Miettinen OS, Williamson JR, Gabbay KH: Muscle capillary basement-membrane thickness and long-term glycemia in type I diabetes mellitus. N Engl J Med 311:694-698, 1984.
11. Engel AG, Tsujihata M, Jerusalem F: Quantitative assessment of motor endplate ultrastructure in normal and diseased human muscle. In Dyck PJ, Thomas PK, Lambert EH, Bunge R (eds): Peripheral Neuropathy, 2nd ed. Philadelphia, Saunders, 1984, pp 871-882.
12. Swash M: Muscle spindle pathology. In Mastaglia FL, Walton JN (eds): Skeletal Muscle Pathology. Edinburgh, Churchill Livingstone, 1982, pp 508-536.
13. Askanas V, Engel WK: Distinct subtypes of type I fibers of human skeletal muscle. Neurology 25:879-887, 1975.
14. Engel WK: Fiber-type nomenclature of human skeletal muscle for histochemical purposes. Neurology 24:344-348, 1974.

chapter 2

Neurogenic Atrophy and Type II Myofiber Atrophy

There are a large number of disorders that injure lower motor neurons or their processes. The resulting changes in the denervated muscle fibers are similar regardless of whether the disease results from the destruction of neuronal perikarya or the disruption of axons. The morphologic variations seen among specimens of skeletal muscle from patients with various denervating conditions reflect the distribution of the injury, i.e., diffuse motor neuron disease versus focal nerve injury, and the tempo of the disease process, i.e., acute, chronic, or remote denervation. Less commonly, denervation results from focal necrosis of muscle fibers so that otherwise intact portions of myofibers are isolated from their neuromuscular junctions. Under these circumstances, myofiber necrosis and inflammatory changes will be conspicuous and may dominate the histopathologic alterations.

The exact factor or factors that are responsible for the morphologic changes in denervated skeletal muscle fibers are not precisely defined. Loss of use, loss of stimulation by quantal releases of acetylcholine, and loss of hypothesized trophic factors have been postulated.[1] The role of acetylcholine seems especially important since there is redistribution of the receptor for this neurotransmitter following denervation. Staining with labeled alpha-bungarotoxin has shown the spread of acetylcholine receptor from the neuromuscular junctions to the entire muscle fiber membrane. In experimental animal models, this commences within a few days of nerve section and persists for up to 6 weeks if reinnervation does not supervene.[2]

MYOFIBER ATROPHY

Regardless of the pathogenesis, the predominant morphologic response to denervation in the adult is progressive atrophy of individual myofibers. The denervated myofibers become shrunken and abnormally angular (Fig. 2–1). In cross-section, the normal rounded to polygonal configuration is lost as the periphery of the myofiber becomes bowed inward. The configurational changes are largely the result of distortion of the shrunken, atrophic fibers by the surrounding normal myofibers. Since a single motor neuron innervates many noncontiguous myofibers in a motor unit, randomly scattered, individual atrophic myofibers are seen when only a few neurons or axons are affected. With progressive involvement of more motor neurons or simultaneous involvement of more axons, small groups of angular atrophic myofibers may be seen (Fig. 2–2). In advanced disease with involvement of many motor neurons or whole peripheral nerves, large groups or fascicles of angular atrophic myofibers may be encountered (Fig. 2–3). Occasionally, when multiple adjacent myofibers undergo atrophy simultaneously, their margins appear scalloped rather than angular.

Nerve section in various laboratory animals produces atrophy that occurs more rapidly and is more severe among the type II myofibers than the type I myofibers. In humans, however, both major fiber types are thought to undergo

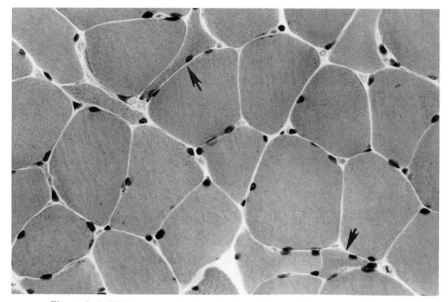

Figure 2–1. Mild neurogenic atrophy in a 60-year-old woman with early amyotrophic lateral sclerosis. Individual denervated fibers *(arrows)* are shrunken and angular in appearance. H&E, ×440.

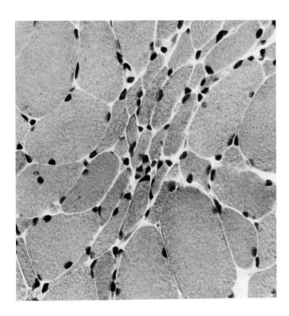

Figure 2-2. Neurogenic atrophy in a 21-year-old woman with weakness and mild atrophy of muscles in the upper limbs. Note the small groups of atrophic angular fibers. H&E, ×410.

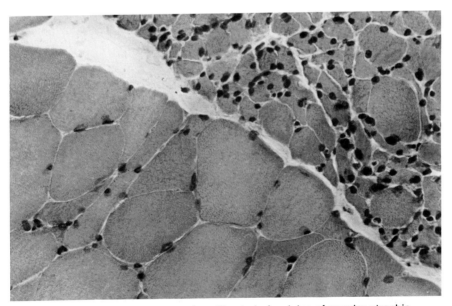

Figure 2-3. Neurogenic atrophy with whole fascicles of angular atrophic fibers *(upper right)*. H&E, ×410.

atrophy approximately at the same rate and to the same degree. Since all denervating diseases affect both type I and type II myofibers, demonstrating that the atrophic myofibers are of both types is essential for the definitive diagnosis of neurogenic atrophy (Fig. 2-4). Fiber typing of the atrophic myofibers can be done reliably only with the ATPase reactions that are relatively resistant to trophic changes. The nonspecific esterase reaction will show increased reactivity (dark staining) in denervated myofibers of either type. This reaction is especially helpful in detecting small numbers of widely scattered, individual denervated myofibers (Fig. 2-5). Atrophic myofibers of both types also stain darkly with the oxidative enzyme stains such as the NADH–TR reaction (Fig. 2-6). This enhanced staining has been attributed to selective loss of contractile elements with relative preservation of mitochondria and other components of the sarcoplasm. By contrast, the myophosphorylase activity and the glycogen content (PAS-positivity) of acutely denervated myofibers are markedly reduced.

Fascicles and small groups of angular atrophic myofibers are readily seen in paraffin-embedded sections and provide reasonably good evidence of denervation even though fiber typing is not possible. It is much more difficult to identify scattered individual atrophic myofibers, and when they are detected, it is virtually impossible to determine whether the atrophy is really neurogenic. Distinguishing common and relatively nonspecific type II myofiber atrophy from neurogenic atrophy is especially difficult. In paraffin-embedded sections, these atrophic myofibers may closely resemble the changes of denervation. Only the widespread distribution of individual atrophic myofibers interposed among normal-sized fibers provides any hint as to the true nature of pathologic change.

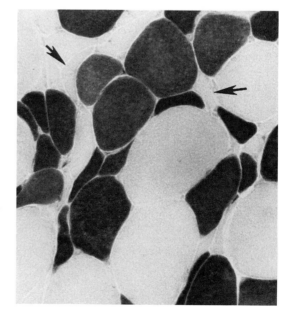

Figure 2-4. The definitive diagnosis of neurogenic atrophy depends on demonstrating that both fiber types are undergoing atrophy. In the ATPase preparation, preincubated at pH 4.2, the atrophic type I myofibers are dark and the atrophic type II myofibers are almost unstained *(arrows)* (same patient shown in Fig. 2-2). ×410.

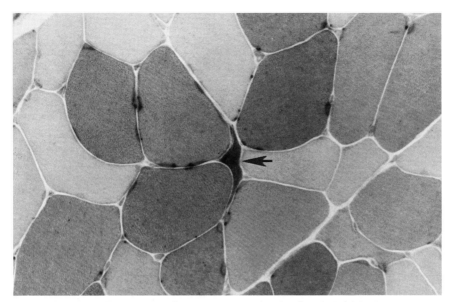

Figure 2-5. The nonspecific esterase reaction is often helpful in detecting small numbers of widely scattered denervated myofibers. Note the single dark-staining denervated myofiber. ×440.

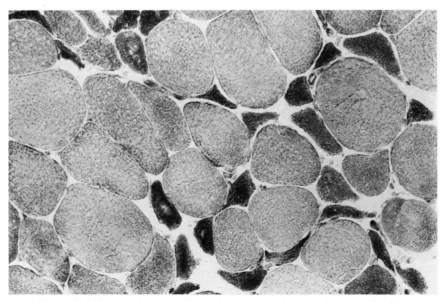

Figure 2-6. Denervated myofibers of both types tend to stain darkly with the NADH-TR reaction. ×220.

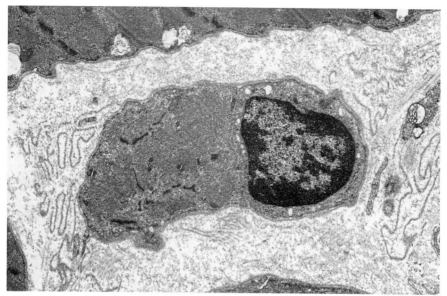

Figure 2-7. This muscle biopsy specimen was from a patient with neuronal Charcot-Marie-Tooth disease. The electron micrograph shows an atrophic myofiber and redundant basement membranes. ×7000.

Eventually denervated myofibers become severely atrophic and appear as clumps of pyknotic nuclei with scanty cytoplasm. Ultrastructural examination discloses folded, redundant surface membranes, relatively large nuclei, and a marked reduction in contractile elements (Fig. 2-7). With the passage of time and no reinnervation, the denervated muscle is largely replaced by fibroadipose tissue. Intrafusal fibers within muscle spindles persist remarkably unchanged. Often the presence of spindles is the only evidence that a specimen of fibroadipose tissue is "end-stage" atrophic muscle rather than merely subcutaneous tissue.

TARGET FIBERS

Target fibers are another pathologic feature that may be encountered in muscle specimens from patients with denervating diseases. This distinctive structural alteration was described in detail by Engel[3] who found them in 27 of 51 biopsy specimens from patients with various neurogenic disorders. The association with denervating diseases has been confirmed on many occasions. Rarely, however, they may be seen in myopathic conditions, especially in the periodic paralyses and inflammatory myopathies. In the latter conditions, they may still be the result of denervation, with myofiber necrosis isolating a portion of a myofiber from the neuromuscular junction. Target fibers were so named because of their distinctive appearance in transverse sections. True target fibers display three concentric rings or zones when cross-sections of the affected myofibers are examined. In humans, the fibers undergoing this alteration are predominantly if not exclusively type I myofibers. Target fibers are seen most clearly in frozen sections stained for oxidative enzyme activity such as with the NADH–TR procedure (Figs. 2–8 and 2–9) and in sections stained for myophosphorylase activity. With these methods, the central zone is pale and devoid of enzyme activity. The intermediate zone is darker and reflects enhanced enzymatic reactivity while the outer peripheral zone shows normal staining. Target fibers are also detected readily with the PAS, trichrome, and ATPase techniques. The central zone stains weakly with the PAS reaction presumably because of the reduced glycogen content of this region. With the trichrome stain, the central region has an abnormally reddish hue as a result of the derangement of the contractile elements. Presumably for the same reasons, the central area often appears unstained with the ATPase reactions. In some cases, target fibers can even be seen with the H&E stain.

In paraffin-embedded sections, target fibers are best seen following the use of the trichrome (Fig. 2–10) or PTAH stains (Fig. 2–11). When seen in longitudinal sections, target formations are found to extend over many sarcomeres but do not extend the whole length of the myofiber. The presence of target fibers is especially helpful in diagnosing neurogenic atrophy from the limited spectrum of changes that can be seen in paraffin-embedded sections.

Target fibers have been studied extensively by electron microscopy.[4-6] The

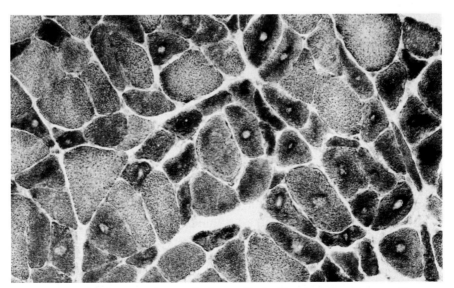

Figure 2-8. Neurogenic atrophy in a patient with a peripheral neuropathy. Note the numerous target fibers, many of which are mildly atrophic type I myofibers. NADH–TR, ×220.

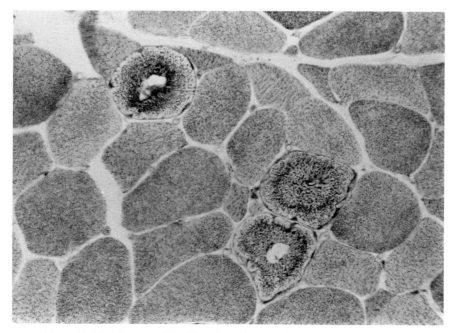

Figure 2-9. Higher-magnification view of target fibers as seen with the NADH-TR reaction. Note the central areas of reduced or no staining, the intermediate zones of enhanced staining, and the peripheral zones of normal staining. ×420.

central zone contains markedly disorganized myofilaments admixed with finely granular, osmiophilic material. This is similar to Z-disc material and appears to be an exaggerated form of Z-disc streaming (Fig. 2–12). Mitochondria and glycogen granules are markedly reduced in number. Cisterns of the sarcoplasmic reticulum and the T-tubules are sparse and disorganized. Small numbers of multivesicular autophagic vacuoles have been described as an additional ultrastructural feature of the central zone of target fibers.[6] The intermediate zone contains thin myofibrils with mild Z-disc streaming and slightly disorganized sarcotubular components. Mitochondria may be increased in number in some instances and are often abnormally small. Glycogen granules may be unusually numerous. The outer zone is generally normal except for mild Z-disc streaming.

Target fibers are encountered most commonly in specimens from patients with peripheral neuropathies. We regard target fibers as reliable evidence of recent active denervation. Target fibers seen in association with chronic peripheral neuropathies may be the result of recurrent episodes of acute denervation. This interpretation is supported by the fact that many of the target fibers are very mildly atrophic. The ultrastructural observations of Mrak et

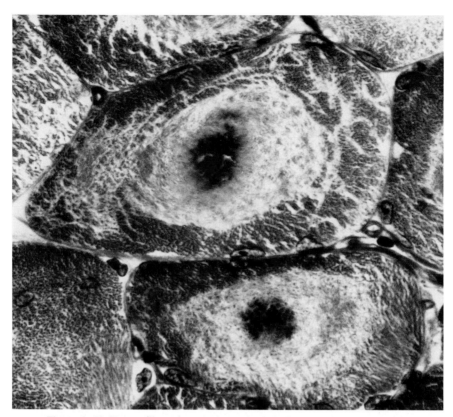

Figure 2-10. Target fibers in a patient who had Guillain-Barré syndrome. The muscle biopsy specimen was fixed in SUSA solution. This paraffin-embedded section was stained by the conventional Gomori trichrome technique. ×800.

al.[6] suggest that target fibers are an involutional or catabolic response to denervation. They further suggest that the pathogenetic events following denervation affect primarily the intermediate zone of the target fibers. The formation of target fibers may be a transient phenomenon. We have observed their development and subsequent disappearance in a patient with Guillain-Barré syndrome.[5] Considering target fibers a manifestation of acute denervation leaves unexplained the failure to demonstrate extrajunctional acetylcholine receptor on the surface of these fibers.[2] Other interpretations also have been put forth. Some authors, including Dubowitz,[7] view target fibers as a manifestation of reinnervation rather than denervation. Morphologically similar changes have been seen in laboratory animals following tenotomy.[8] However, these alterations might be better interpreted as targetoid or core-targetoid fibers that are related to alterations in muscular activity.

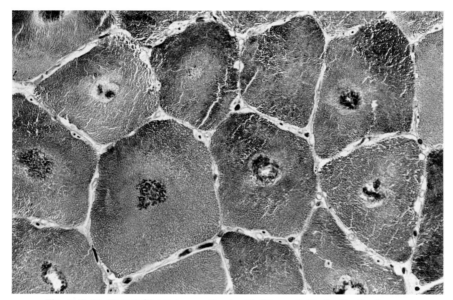

Figure 2-11. Target fibers in a patient with Charcot–Marie–Tooth disease. The muscle biopsy was fixed in SUSA solution. The paraffin-embedded section was stained with PTAH. ×550.

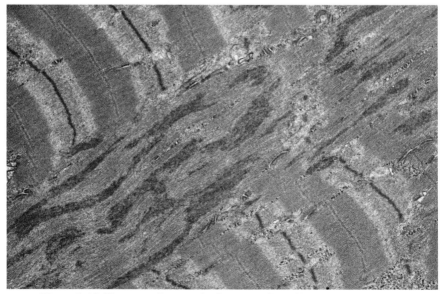

Figure 2-12. Electron micrograph of a target fiber. Note the central area of myofibrillar disarray. ×5000.

TARGETOID FIBERS

Targetoid fibers differ from target fibers in as much as they lack the intermediate region and thus have only two zones. They are less specific evidence of denervation and have been encountered in a wide variety of neurogenic and myopathic disorders. They closely resemble the central cores found in central core disease, one of the so-called congenital myopathies. Because of the morphologic similarities, the term "core-targetoid" fibers has been proposed to describe these fibers.

SECONDARY MYOPATHIC CHANGES

Chronic partial denervation, especially when accompanied by persistent functional overload, may lead to the development of gross and histologic changes that are associated more commonly with myopathies. This is illustrated dramatically by examples of calf hypertrophy that have been reported in association with relatively benign forms of motor neuron disease, radiculopathies, and neuropathies.[9-11] The histologic changes that occur against a background of chronic neurogenic disease are often designated as "secondary myopathic" changes (Fig. 2-13). Some of the muscle fibers, especially type I myofibers, may hypertrophy and contain increased numbers of internal nuclei. Fissures may develop between the internal nuclei and the surface of the myofiber. The sarcoplasm adjacent to the fissures often stains darkly and contains excessive glycogen, ribosomes, mitochondria, and myofibrillar debris.[12] Ultimately the portions of the myofiber divided by the fissure separate, a process known as fiber splitting. Although this mechanism is widely accepted to explain the fiber splitting associated with persistent mechanical overload, alternative mechanisms have been proposed for fiber splitting in other situations. These include reinnervation of denervated myofibers, activation of satellite cells in the absence of necrosis, and incomplete fusion of myoblasts following muscle necrosis.[13]

Rare necrotic myofibers may be encountered as another of the nonspecific, "secondary myopathic" changes. The necrotic fibers may elicit or are at least accompanied by mild interstitial or perivascular inflammatory cell infiltrates. Changes may be seen among the endomysial capillaries. With atrophy and loss of myofiber volume, capillaries become more closely approximated and increased in number per unit area. At the same time, however, Carpenter and Karpati have shown that some of the capillaries in denervated muscle undergo necrosis.[14] Jerusalem[15] described a reduced capillary density among hypertrophied muscle fibers in patients with chronic neurogenic atrophy. Capillaries may be found in the depths of the clefts produced by fiber splitting. In addition, we have seen "internalized capillaries," capillaries that appear to be coursing through the interior of muscle fibers, in association with chronic partial denervation. Although internalized capillaries are rarely encountered they

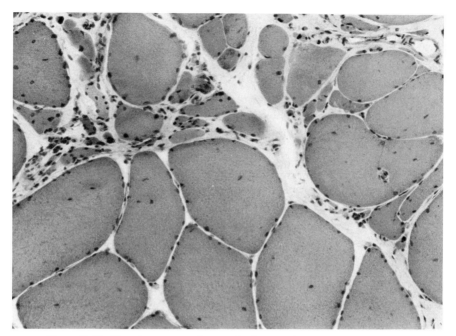

Figure 2-13. Chronic neurogenic atrophy in a patient with benign amyotrophy. Note the hypertrophied myofibers, split myofibers, and increased numbers of internal nuclei along with small groups of angular atrophic myofibers. H&E, × 175.

have been observed in association with diverse disorders including neuropathies, Becker dystrophy, and hypokalemic periodic paralysis.[16-18] Internalized capillaries are found more often within type I myofibers than type II myofibers. Since the internalized capillaries often appear paired (Fig. 2–14), we have suggested that they represent deep invaginations of myofibers by proliferating capillary loops. These probably arise from capillaries contained within the clefts of split myofibers.

With further progression of the neurogenic atrophy and passage of time, there is proliferation of endomysial and perimysial connective tissue. Eventually the muscle becomes replaced by fibroadipose tissue with only occasional muscle spindles remaining to identify its origin.

FIBER TYPE GROUPING

All of the muscle fibers within a single motor unit are of the same fiber type. These histochemical properties are determined by the lower motor neuron that innervates them. Muscle fibers belonging to different motor units, however, are normally intermingled. Thus, normal skeletal muscle is a random mosaic

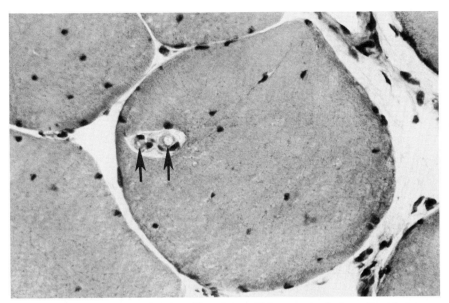

Figure 2-14. Internalized capillary loop within a markedly hypertrophied myofiber from a patient with chronic neurogenic atrophy. Note the two lumens *(arrows)*. H&E, ×440.

of different fiber types. Following denervation, acetylcholine receptor spreads from the myoneural junction over the surface of the denervated myofiber. Under these conditions, the myofibers can be reinnervated by axonal sprouts from nearby intact nerve fibers. Since the fiber type is determined by the nature of the motor neuron, the reinnervation results in a group of adjacent muscle fibers becoming transformed to a single fiber type. This process is referred to as "fiber type grouping." Although fiber type grouping is virtually pathognomonic of denervating diseases, the process is actually a manifestation of reinnervation. Recognition of fiber type grouping depends on stains that identify the fiber types and is best seen in sections stained by the ATPase (Fig. 2–15) or NADH–TR (Fig. 2–16) reactions. The phenomenon generally cannot be detected in paraffin-embedded sections. The minimum number of fibers of the same type that must be present in the groups is undetermined. Some workers arbitrarily consider only groups of 13 or more fibers to be significant. Karpati et al.[19] have described small groups of a single fiber type resulting from regeneration, so-called "myopathic fiber type grouping." However, when there is fiber type predominance, groups composed of only a few fibers of the minority type may be considered evidence of reinnervation.[20] Groups composed of only one of the two major fiber types are a less reliable indicator of reinnervation since they may result from fiber type predominance.

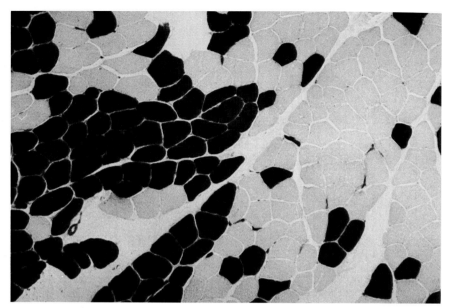

Figure 2-15. Fiber type grouping secondary to reinnervation in a patient with a polyneuropathy. The type I myofibers are stained darkly in this preparation. ATPase following preincubation at pH 4.2, ×100.

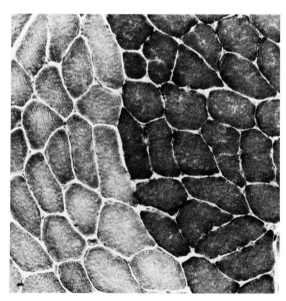

Figure 2-16. Fiber type grouping secondary to reinnervation in a patient with Kugelberg–Welander disease. The type I myofibers are stained darkly in this preparation. NADH–TR, ×175.

NEUROGENIC ATROPHY IN INFANCY AND CHILDHOOD

Denervation of skeletal muscle in infancy produces histopathologic changes that are different from those seen in the adult. These differences are especially marked in muscle specimens from patients with the severe (type I) and intermediate (type II) forms of infantile spinal muscular atrophy. By contrast, the changes seen in the mild juvenile (type III) spinal muscular atrophy closely resemble the changes of chronic neurogenic atrophy in the adult. Whether the severe (type I), intermediate (type II), and mild (type III) forms of spinal muscular atrophy are distinct diseases or merely age-related variants of the same disorder, remains controversial. All appear to be inherited as autosomal-recessive disorders.

The severe and intermediate forms are often considered together as Werdnig–Hoffmann disease. This disease has an incidence of about 4/100,000 individuals. The clinical manifestations of the severe form are often evident at birth or become evident during the first 6 months of life. In about one third of the cases, the mothers report decreased intrauterine movements suggesting prenatal onset of the disease. The clinical manifestations in the infants with the intermediate form generally become evident between the ages of 6 and 12 months. In both groups, the major manifestations include weakness, hypotonia, and areflexia. The lower limbs are more severely affected than the upper limbs and the muscles innervated by cranial nerves are generally spared. These diseases are major considerations in the differential diagnosis of the so-called "floppy infant."

The pathogenesis of these diseases is commonly attributed to the degeneration of motor neurons in the spinal cord and to a lesser extent, the brain stem. Alternatively, Chou et al.[21,22] have suggested that the primary insult may affect the motor nerve roots where it produces proliferation of glia. They regard the chromatolysis and neuronal degeneration as secondary to the glial hyperplasia. More recently, it has been suggested that the glial bundles in the ventral roots are a nonspecific epiphenomenon since they also have been seen in cases of poliomyelitis, amyotrophic lateral sclerosis, and other neurogenic processes.[23,24] Furthermore, other authors have suggested that the neurodegenerative changes in Werdnig–Hoffmann disease may not be confined to the motor neurons and their processes.[25] Degenerative changes have been documented in the thalamus, dorsal root ganglia, and peripheral sensory nerves.[23,25] Some of these cases may be considered as examples of the more recently delineated condition, infantile neuronal degeneration.[26]

Even among infants with the severe form of infantile spinal muscular atrophy, there is variation in the histopathology of skeletal muscle depending upon the age of the infant and the stage of the disease. Specimens from infants less than 1 month of age may show only mild myofiber atrophy that is somewhat more severe among the type I myofibers. Dubowitz[27] has designated this condition as the "prepathological" stage. Specimens from infants who have the severe form of spinal muscular atrophy and are more than 1 month of age generally show fascicles and large groups of highly atrophic myofibers. The atrophic myofibers are of both types but in contrast to those found in the adult, the atrophic myofibers in infants often appear rounded rather than angular (Figs. 2–17 and 2–18). Frequently the atrophic myofibers are so small that the nuclei appear internal in location. A few fibers may even appear to contain true central nuclei. In addition to the atrophic fibers, there are characteristically groups of very large myofibers which may measure up to 80 μm in diameter. These large myofibers are predominantly but not exclusively type I myofibers as judged by their reaction with the ATPase procedures (Fig. 2–19). Staining with other techniques, especially the oxidative enzyme stains, gives varied results. The pathogenesis of these large fibers remains undetermined. Some authors have regarded them as persistent Wohlfart type b fibers while others interpret their development as the result of compensatory work hypertrophy among reinnervated myofibers.[28] Sarnat[29] has made the observation that unlike other diseases of infancy, large numbers of the myofibers stain with the alkaline phosphatase reaction. Other histopathologic changes that are commonly seen in denervation, such as pyknotic nuclei and target fibers, are conspicuously absent. The quantity of endomysial connective tissue and especially, the quantity of perimysial connective tissue appears increased. Muscle spindles may be encountered with increased frequency but this is probably due to the predominant atrophy of the extrafusal fibers. Many of these changes can be seen in paraffin-embedded sections. However, the characteristic atrophy of both

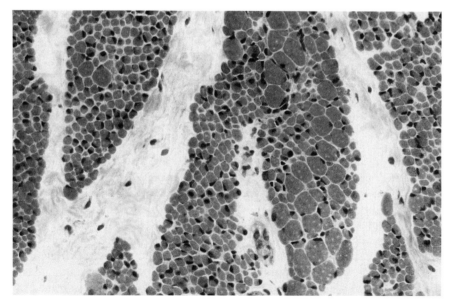

Figure 2-17. Muscle biopsy specimen from a "floppy infant" with Werdnig–Hoffmann disease. Note the rounded atrophic myofibers and small groups of normal-sized to hypertrophied myofibers. H&E, ×220.

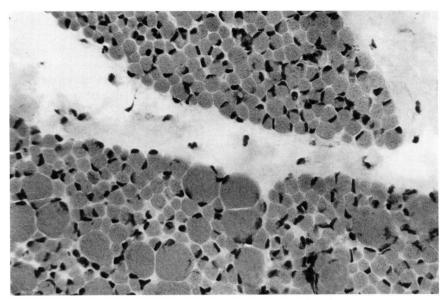

Figure 2-18. Muscle biopsy specimen from another infant with Werdnig-Hoffmann disease. Some of the atrophic myofibers are so small that the nuclei spuriously appear "internalized." H&E, ×440.

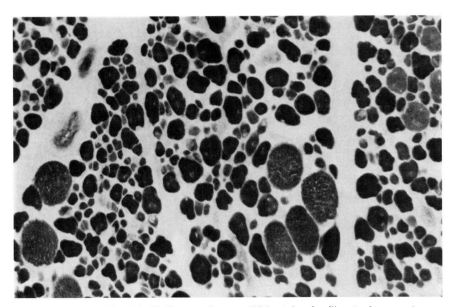

Figure 2-19. Werdnig-Hoffmann disease. With stains for fiber typing, most of the hypertrophied fibers stain as type I myofibers (lighter with this stain). ATPase, pH 9.4, ×440.

fiber types and the hypertrophy, predominantly of type I myofibers, cannot be appreciated.

Muscle specimens from children with the mild juvenile (type III) spinal muscular atrophy or Kugelberg–Welander disease show changes that are similar to the changes of chronic denervation and reinnervation in the adult. Fiber type grouping and large group atrophy with prominent secondary myopathic changes may be seen.

TYPE II MYOFIBER ATROPHY

Type II myofiber atrophy is a very commonly encountered pathologic change in muscle specimens. It can be seen readily both in paraffin-embedded sections and in frozen sections stained with H&E, trichrome, and so forth. Under these conditions, one often sees large numbers of moderately atrophic myofibers intermixed randomly with normal-sized fibers. However, accurate identification of this process can be made only in frozen sections appropriately stained for fiber typing, especially with the ATPase reactions (Fig. 2–20). Type II myofibers, especially type IIB myofibers, are subject to atrophy in a wide variety of conditions. These include various neurodegenerative disorders, myasthenia gravis, collagen–vascular diseases, neoplastic diseases, disuse, Cushing's disease, and iatrogenic steroid myopathy. Although type II myofibers atrophy more

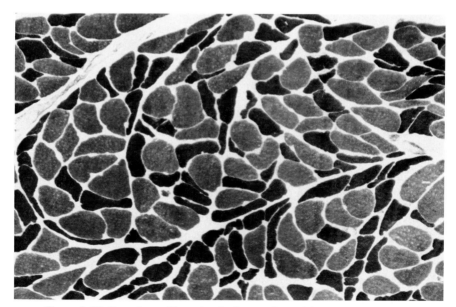

Figure 2-20. Type II myofiber atrophy in a patient with systemic amyloidosis. Note the widespread selective atrophy of the dark-staining type II myofibers. ATPase, pH 9.4, ×175.

rapidly than type I myofibers following nerve section in experimental animals, type II myofiber atrophy is not particularly associated with denervating diseases in humans. The small fibers seen in type II myofiber atrophy do not consistently stain darkly with the NADH–TR or the nonspecific esterase reactions. Furthermore, histochemical studies have not shown spread of extrajunctional acetylcholine receptors on the surface of the atrophic myofibers as in neurogenic atrophy.[2] Thus it would appear that there are fundamental differences between the type II myofiber atrophy following experimental neurotomy in laboratory animals and the type II myofiber atrophy seen so commonly in muscle specimens in human diseases.

References

1. Engel WK: Introduction to disorders of the motor neuron, nerves and related abnormalities. In Goldensohn ES, Appel SH (eds): Scientific Approaches to Clinical Neurology. Philadelphia, Lea & Febiger, 1977, Vol. 2, pp 1250–1321.
2. Ringel SP, Bender AN, Engel WK: Extrajunctional acetylcholine receptors. Alterations in human and experimental neuromuscular diseases. Arch Neurol 33:751–758, 1976.
3. Engel WK: Muscle target fibers, a newly recognized sign of denervation. Nature 191:389–390, 1961.
4. DeCoster W, DeReuck J, Van der Eecken H: The target phenomenon in human muscle: A comparative light microscopic and electron microscopic study. Acta Neuropathol 34:329–338, 1976.
5. Kovarsky J, Schochet SS Jr, McCormick WF: The significance of target fibers: A clinicopathologic review of 100 patients with neurogenic atrophy. Am J Clin Pathol 59:790–797, 1973.
6. Mrak RE, Akitsugu S, Evans OB, Fleischer S: Autophagic degradation in human skeletal muscle target fibers. Muscle Nerve 5:745–753, 1982.
7. Dubowitz V: Pathology of experimentally re-innervated skeletal muscle. J Neurol Neurosurg Psychiatry 30:99–110, 1967.
8. DeReuck J, DeCoster W, Van der Eecken H: The target phenomenon in rat muscle following tenotomy and neurotomy. Acta Neuropathol 37:49–53, 1977.
9. D'Alessandro R, Montagna P, Govoni E, Pazzaglia P: Benign familial spinal muscular atrophy with hypertrophy of the calves. Arch Neurol 39:657–660, 1982.
10. Montagna P, Martinelli P, Rasi F, et al.: Muscular hypertrophy after chronic radiculopathy. Arch Neurol 41:397–398, 1982.
11. Riggs JE, Schochet SS Jr, Gutmann L: Benign focal amyotrophy. Variant of chronic spinal muscular atrophy. Arch Neurol 41:678–679, 1984.
12. Schwartz MS, Sargeant M, Swash M: Longitudinal fibre splitting in neurogenic muscular disorders—Its relation to the pathogenesis of "myopathic" change. Brain 99:617–636, 1976.
13. Carpenter S, Karpati G: Pathology of Skeletal Muscle. New York, Churchill Livingstone, 1984, pp 125–128.
14. Carpenter S, Karpati G: Necrosis of capillaries in denervation atrophy of human skeletal muscle. Muscle Nerve 5:250–254, 1982.
15. Jerusalem F: Circulatory disorders and pathology of intramuscular blood vessels. In

Mastaglia FL, Walton JN (eds): Skeletal Muscle Pathology. Edinburgh, Churchill Livingstone, 1982, pp 537–560.

16. Hastings BA, Groothuis DR, Vick NA: Dominantly inherited pseudohypertrophic muscular dystrophy with internalized capillaries. Arch Neurol 37:709–714, 1980.

17. Schmitt HP: Internalized capillaries. Arch Neurol 38:602, 1981.

18. Hartlage PL, Soudmand R: Internalized capillaries in hypokalemic periodic paralysis. Arch Neurol 38:602, 1981.

19. Karpati G, Carpenter S, Melmed C, Eisen AA: Experimental ischemic myopathy. J Neurol Sci 23:129–161, 1974.

20. Jennekens FGI: Neurogenic disorders of muscle. In Mastaglia FL, Walton JN (eds): Skeletal Muscle Pathology. Edinburgh, Churchill Livingstone, 1982, pp 204–234.

21. Chou SM, Fakadej AV: Ultrastructure of chromatolytic motor neurons and anterior spinal roots in a case of Werdnig–Hoffmann disease. J Neuropathol Exp Neurol 30:368–379, 1971.

22. Chou SM, Nonaka I: Werdnig–Hoffmann disease: Proposal of a pathogenetic mechanism. Acta Neuropathol 41:45–54, 1978.

23. Iwata M, Hirano A: "Glial bundles" in the spinal cord late after paralytic poliomyelitis. Ann Neurol 4:562–563, 1978.

24. Ghatak NR, Nochlin D: Glial outgrowth along spinal nerve roots in amyotrophic lateral sclerosis. Ann Neurol 11:203–206, 1982.

25. Carpenter S, Karpati G, Rothman S, et al.: Pathological involvement of primary sensory neurons in Werdnig–Hoffmann disease. Acta Neuropathol 42:91–97, 1978.

26. Steiman GS, Rorke LB, Brown MJ: Infantile neuronal degeneration masquerading as Werdnig–Hoffmann disease. Ann Neurol 8:317–324, 1980.

27. Dubowitz V: Muscle Disorders in Childhood. London, Saunders, 1978, p 169.

28. Dubowitz V, Brooke MH: Muscle Biopsy: A Modern Approach. London, Saunders, 1973, p 155.

29. Sarnat HB: Muscle Pathology and Histochemistry. Chicago, American Society of Clinical Pathologists, 1983, p 40.

chapter 3

Inflammatory Myopathies

INTRODUCTION AND CLASSIFICATION

The inflammatory myopathies encompass a large group of diverse disorders. Some are relatively common diseases while others are quite rare. They can be divided readily into two unequal groups, the so-called idiopathic inflammatory myopathies and a smaller, more heterogeneous group of disorders caused by specific, identifiable etiologic agents. Further classification, especially of the idiopathic inflammatory myopathies, is controversial. Many of the published classifications, based primarily on clinical criteria, categorize the idiopathic inflammatory myopathies according to the patient's age and the presence or absence of associated skin lesions, connective tissue disease, or malignancies.[1-3] Some workers regard polymyositis and dermatomyositis as variants of the same disorder[4] while others maintain that they are distinct entities. For the purpose of this discussion, we will emphasize differential morphologic criteria and will employ a classification (Table 3-1) that is similar to the one proposed by Carpenter and Karpati.[5]

Many workers regard the idiopathic inflammatory myopathies as immunologically mediated disorders. This interpretation is supported by the increased prevalence of these diseases in association with other immunologic disorders, the favorable therapeutic response that is often obtained with immunosuppressive therapy and certain experimental models.[6] It is further supported by various immunohistochemical studies on biopsy specimens from patients with these diseases. Abnormal deposits of immunoglobulins have been demonstrated in intramuscular vessel walls and interstitial tissue by several groups of investigators.[7-10] The more recent studies have attempted to determine the nature of the inflammatory cells. The cellular infiltrates have been analyzed with regard to the relative proportions of B cells, subtypes of T cells, and macrophages. Arahata and Engel[11] found the endomysial inflammatory cell infiltrates in polymyositis and inclusion body myositis to consist predominantly of T cells and macrophages. By contrast, they found a higher percentage of B

TABLE 3-1. INFLAMMATORY MYOPATHIES

IDIOPATHIC INFLAMMATORY MYOPATHY
  Polymyositis
  Juvenile dermatomyositis
  Adult dermatomyositis
  Inclusion body myositis

INFLAMMATORY MYOPATHIES ASSOCIATED
  WTIH CONNECTIVE TISSUE DISEASE
  Scleroderma
  Lupus erythematosus
  Rheumatoid disease
  Sjögren's syndrome
  Polyarteritis
  Eosinophilic myositis

MISCELLANEOUS INFLAMMATORY MYOPATHIES
  Focal and granulomatous myositis
  Bacterial myositis
  Fungal myositis
  Parasitic myositis
  Viral myositis

FACTITIOUS MYOSITIS

cells, especially within the perivascular inflammatory cell infiltrates in dermatomyositis.

Although viruses have been implicated in certain forms of acute and subacute myositis,[3] there is little evidence for their involvement in the usual chronic inflammatory myopathies. Certain ultrastructural findings that have been purported to support a viral etiology for these disorders, are subject to other interpretations. Some of the abnormal structures such as small dense particles resembling virions, might also be interpreted as postmortem artifacts[12-14] or glycogen deposits.[15] The myxoviruslike filaments[16-20] characteristically seen in inclusion body myositis are probably altered myofilament proteins rather than the etiologic agent. Other structures demonstrated by electron microscopy, such as the undulating tubular arrays in dermatomyositis, are probably important indicators of cellular injury but are not viral in nature.[21,22] Only rarely have viruses actually been isolated from the muscle of patients with inflammatory myopathy. Even in these cases, the serious question remains as to whether the viruses are coincidentally present or are the actual etiologic agents.[15,20,23]

Polymyositis

Although polymyositis can occur at any age, it is seen most often in adults. In most series, women are affected more commonly than men. The disease usually progresses gradually over a period of weeks to months. Occasionally, there are spontaneous relapses and remissions. Weakness, especially of the proximal limb muscles and the neck flexors, is a cardinal manifestation of the disease. Many of the patients also have pain, tenderness, and swelling in the affected muscles. Dysphagia is another fairly common symptom. The serum muscle enzymes such as CK are generally elevated during the course of active disease but may decline with remission. Electromyography generally discloses a mixture of fibrillations and brief, small amplitude, polyphasic potentials.

Muscle specimens from patients with polymyositis commonly show increased variation in myofiber size (Figs. 3–1 and 3–2). This variation is due predominantly to the presence of mildly atrophic myofibers. The atrophic fibers are scattered randomly or aggregated in ill-defined groups but do not show the distinctive perifascicular localization that is characteristic of dermatomyositis. The atrophic myofibers are usually of both major fiber types. Occasionally, they are predominantly type II fibers, however, this may be the result of concurrent type II atrophy from disuse or steroid therapy. The atrophic fibers tend to be rounded and do not show the sharp angularity that is more characteristic of neurogenic atrophy. There is usually little myofiber hypertrophy. This is an important feature for distinguishing chronic myositis from some of the dystrophies, e.g., facioscapulohumeral dystrophy, that may be accompanied by inflammatory cell infiltrates.

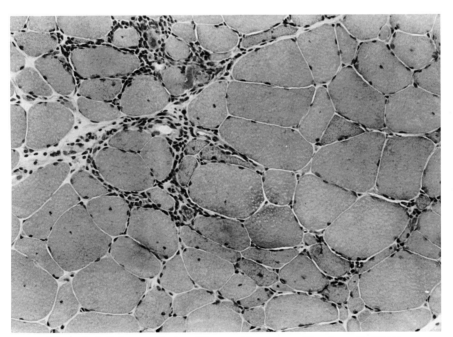

Figure 3-1. Polymyositis in a 68-year-old woman with a 6-month history of progressive weakness of proximal limb and neck muscles. The specimen shows increased variation in myofiber size, a small number of degenerating and regenerating myofibers, and focal mononuclear inflammatory cell infiltrates. Trichrome, ×220.

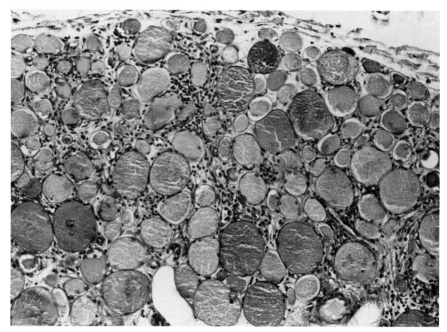

Figure 3-2. Polymyositis in a 43-year-old woman with marked proximal limb muscle weakness and tenderness. This paraffin-embedded section shows marked variation in myofiber size, scattered degenerating myofibers, and prominent mononuclear inflammatory cell infiltrates. PAS, ×220.

A wide variety of relatively nonspecific degenerative changes may be seen in the myofibers. Some of the fibers have irregular smudgy areas that stain abnormally blue with H&E and reddish purple with the trichrome technique. These areas of altered staining are the result of myofibrillary disarray and Z-disc streaming. When especially severe, these derangements can result in fibers that have large central areas that are darkly stained with the NADH–TR reaction (Fig. 3–3) and weakly if at all with the ATPase reaction. The Z-disc alterations in cases of polymyositis are generally less pronounced than in cases of dermatomyositis. Occasionally cytoplasmic bodies are encountered. These are small rounded masses that stain red with the trichrome technique and are surrounded by a lighter-staining halo. They also may be seen in paraffin- and epoxy-embedded sections (Fig. 3–4). By electron microscopy, cytoplasmic bodies appear to be composed of a core of fine granular material surrounded by a peripheral band of fine filaments (Fig. 3–5). They are encountered predominantly in type II myofibers and are probably derived from Z-disc material.[24] Cytoplasmic bodies are a nonspecific finding and may be seen in other disorders.

In some cases of acute polymyositis, clear vacuoles may be seen. These are

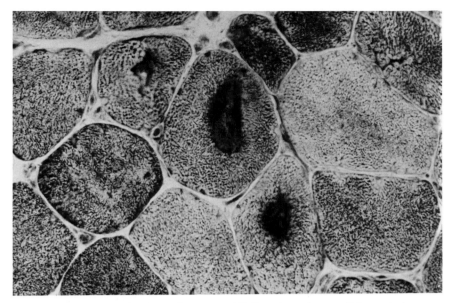

Figure 3-3. Myofibrillary disarray and Z-disc streaming result in central areas that stain abnormally dark with the NADH–TR reaction. ×400.

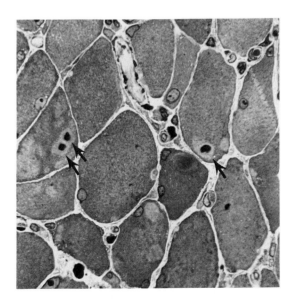

Figure 3-4. Cytoplasmic bodies *(arrows)* as seen in an epoxy-embedded section stained with toluidine blue. Although cytoplasmic bodies may be encountered in polymyositis, they are a nonspecific alteration. ×600.

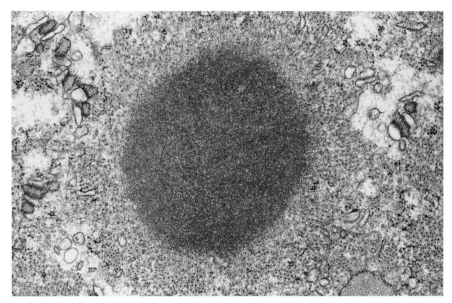

Figure 3-5. Electron micrograph of a cytoplasmic body. Note the granular center and surrounding filaments. ×80,000.

either autophagic vacuoles or the result of marked dilatation of cisterns of the sarcoplasmic reticulum or T-tubules. Rarefied areas may be seen at the periphery of some of the myofibers. These result from lysis of peripherally situated myofibrils followed by nonspecific accumulation of glycogen. In more chronic cases, fiber splitting, whorled fibers, and even nemaline rods may be seen. The number of internal nuclei may be increased markedly. Although these nuclei are usually unremarkable except for their location, small intranuclear inclusions have been encountered in some patients.[25] Ultrastructurally they are composed of fine filaments (Fig. 3-6). These have been variously interpreted as being derived from nuclear bodies or as actin filaments that have polymerized from globular actin that has diffused into the nucleus. The fine filaments that comprise these inclusions are readily distinguished by electron microscopy from the coarse filaments that are characteristic of inclusion body myopathy (see below).

A variable number of necrotic myofibers may be scattered randomly or clustered in small groups. The necrotic fibers often stain abnormally pale and appear "liquefied" (Fig. 3-7). The necrotic sarcoplasm becomes invaded by mononuclear phagocytes; this is so-called "myophagocytosis." In longitudinal sections, the necrosis is found to be segmental, i.e., only portions of the myofiber are affected. Furthermore, the necrosis and myophagocytosis may be more extensive in the center of a fiber than at the periphery. Therefore, in cross-section, one may see apparently intact sarcoplasm surrounding cores of necrotic sarcoplasm, clusters of phagocytes, or both (Fig. 3-8). Eventually all

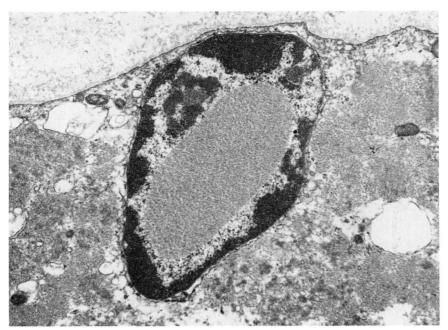

Figure 3-6. Occasionally specimens from patients with polymyositis contain intranuclear inclusions that are composed of thin filaments. These must be distinguished from the thicker filaments that are characteristic of inclusion body myositis. ×30,000.

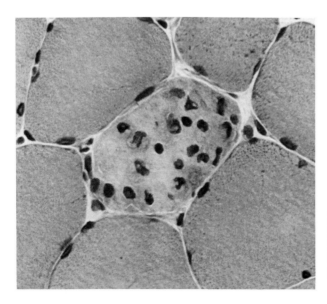

Figure 3-7. Necrotic, liquefied-appearing myofiber that is being invaded by mononuclear phagocytes. Trichrome, ×410.

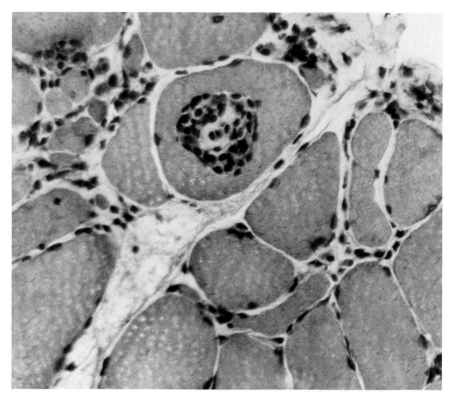

Figure 3-8. Because the necrosis and myophagocytosis are segmental and more severe in the center of the myofiber, one may occasionally see focal collections of phagocytes that appear to be surrounded by intact sarcoplasm. H&E, ×410.

of the sarcoplasm undergoes necrosis and only the basement membrane surrounds a cluster of phagocytes where a myofiber formerly had been (Fig. 3–9). The macrophagic infiltrates can be dramatically highlighted by the use of the nonspecific esterase stain. With this technique, the phagocytic cells stain dark brown against the yellow to brown background of muscle fibers. The persisting basement membranes facilitate regeneration by providing guidance for myoblasts derived from activated satellite cells. Regeneration can occur concurrently with the necrosis and phagocytosis. The regenerating myofibers or portions of myofibers can be recognized by their amphophilic cytoplasm and large vesicular nuclei. They are further characterized by their staining with the alkaline phosphatase reaction. By electron microscopy, the regenerating cells display numerous free ribosomes and randomly oriented filaments.

Although inflammation is a cardinal feature for the histologic diagnosis of polymyositis, its extent is highly variable. The inflammatory cells, whether scanty or abundant, are found in the endomysial connective tissue as well as

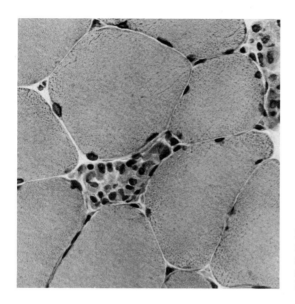

Figure 3-9. Eventually only a basement membrane surrounding a group of phagocytes indicates where a necrotic myofiber had been. H&E, ×410.

about blood vessels. The inflammatory cells can be found around apparently intact myofibers[26] as well as near necrotic fibers. Carpenter and Karpati[5] have described an inflammatory degenerative process called "partial invasion" that they regard as a common finding in polymyositis. The fibers affected by this alteration are not necrotic but appear to have their cytoplasm displaced by mononuclear cells that have insinuated themselves beneath an intact plasmalemma (Fig. 3-10). On the basis of ultrastructural findings, these authors have suggested that inflammatory cells may invade otherwise intact myofibers by way of enlarged T-tubule orifices. However, because of the segmental nature of the myofiber necrosis and phagocytosis, we have great difficulty distinguishing this process of "partial invasion" from the periphery of a necrotic focus.

Lymphocytes and macrophages are the principal inflammatory cells encountered in polymyositis. Recently the lymphocytes have been shown to be predominantly T cells.[11] Rarely, plasma cells may be numerous. These are most often encountered in the perimysial connective tissue, and especially when the inflammatory myopathy is associated with other connective tissue diseases such as lupus erythematosus, rheumatoid disease, scleroderma, and Sjögren's syndrome. In acute and early cases of polymyositis, the endomysial connective tissue often appears edematous, while in the more chronic cases it undergoes progressive fibrosis. The endomysial and perimysial blood vessels may show increased reactivity with the alkaline phosphatase reaction. In contrast to childhood dermatomyositis, capillaries are not significantly reduced in number, however, they may show duplication of basement membranes.[27] Occasionally small foci of neurogenic atrophy are encountered in specimens from patients with otherwise typical polymyositis. These are variously regarded as the result

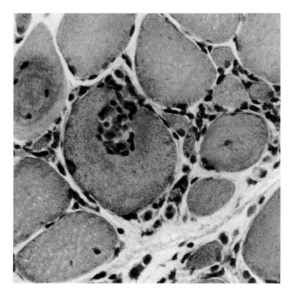

Figure 3-10. Mononuclear cells appear to have penetrated beneath the plasmalemma of an intact myofiber. This process, referred to as "partial invasion,"[5] might also be interpreted as the result of segmental necrosis and phagocytosis. H&E, ×410.

of extension of the inflammation to involve small intramuscular nerve twigs or as the result of denervation of parts of myofibers isolated from the neuromuscular junctions by severe segmental necrosis.

Dermatomyositis

About one third of all patients with idiopathic inflammatory myopathy develop skin lesions. The presence of these cutaneous lesions is the main clinical feature that distinguishes dermatomyositis from polymyositis. Dermatomyositis occurs in both adults and children. In some patients, the skin lesions may appear before the other manifestations of the disease become evident.[28] The skin lesions are varied. Among the more typical cutaneous alterations are a heliotrope discoloration of the upper eyelids; an erythematous rash over the malar eminences, neck, and chest; a scaling erythematous rash over the extensor surfaces of the elbows, knuckles, and knees; there is periungual hyperemia; and a shiny atrophic appearance of the skin over the fingertips is seen. In rare chronic cases, especially in children, there may be subcutaneous mineral deposits, the so-called "calcinosis cutis."

Other than the skin changes, the clinical manifestations of dermatomyositis are similar to those of polymyositis. The limb weakness and dysphagia may develop more rapidly in some patients. In some of the childhood cases, the skin and muscle lesions may be accompanied by systemic vasculitis. In these patients involvement of the gastrointestinal tract may lead to ischemic necrosis, intestinal perforations, and gastrointestinal hemorrhages.[29]

Muscle specimens from patients with dermatomyositis show increased variation in myofiber size. This may be of a morphologically distinctive type. Specimens from almost all children and at least some adults with dermatomyositis show perifascicular atrophy. This alteration is characterized by the presence of atrophic myofibers of both types that are localized along the periphery of scattered fascicles of muscle (Figs. 3–11 and 3–12). The affected fascicles are often adjacent to broad bands of perimysial connective tissue. This is a highly characteristic alteration, and in some specimens, it may be the only morphologic evidence of the disease. Occasionally, small fascicles will be composed almost completely of mildly to moderately atrophic myofibers. Specimens from adults with dermatomyositis may show random variation in myofiber size as well as perifascicular atrophy. A few patients with inflammatory myopathy show perifascicular atrophy without obvious skin lesions.

A wide spectrum of degenerative myofiber alterations may be seen in dermatomyositis. Many of the myofibers in and about the areas of perifascicular atrophy stain abnormally blue with H&E and abnormally reddish with the trichrome technique. These tinctorial alterations are due to extensive Z-disc streaming. In addition, the atrophic fibers frequently stain unevenly and excessively darkly with the NADH–TR reaction. Other fibers, often ones that are not atrophic but adjacent to the regions of perifascicular atrophy, show large central areas of dark staining with the NADH–TR reaction. These fibers resemble targetoid fibers and are further characterized by a focal lack of ATPase reactivity. This alteration has been attributed to lysis of contractile elements. Some myofibers harbor vacuoles containing lipid and glycogen (Fig. 3–13).

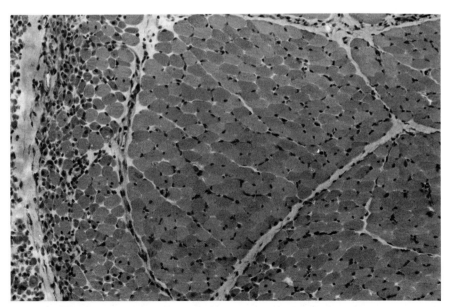

Figure 3-11. Dermatomyositis in a 3-year-old boy with muscle weakness. Note the striking perifascicular atrophy *(left)* with minimal inflammatory cell infiltrates. H&E, × 175.

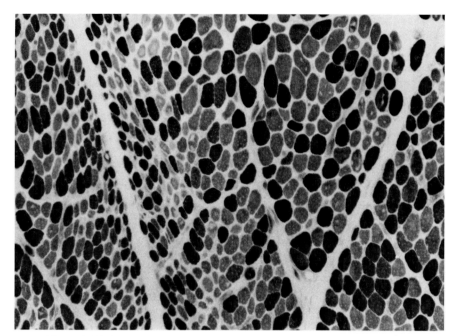

Figure 3–12. Dermatomyositis in a 7-year-old boy with a 2-month history of progressive muscle weakness. He had a rash about his eyes and over his knuckles, elbows, and knees. Fibers showing perifascicular atrophy are of both major types. ATPase, pH 10.4, ×175.

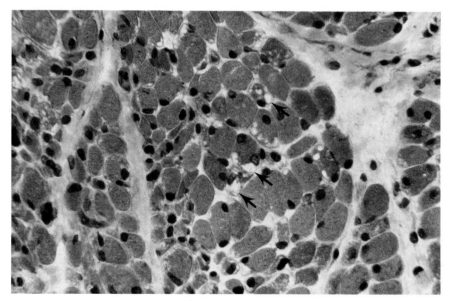

Figure 3–13. Some of the atrophic myofibers are locally vacuolated *(arrows)*, H&E. ×410.

Other nonspecific alterations such as cytoplasmic bodies, nemaline rods, whorled fibers, and ring fibers may be seen in variable numbers.

Necrotic fibers are generally scanty in specimens from children with dermatomyositis but may be more numerous in specimens from adults with dermatomyositis. When present in cases of childhood dermatomyositis, the necrotic fibers are often confined to small groups in which the fibers appear excessively eosinophilic or even vacuolated. These lesions have been interpreted as areas of microinfarction. In adults with dermatomyositis, the necrotic myofibers occur both in groups and widely scattered as in polymyositis. The inflammatory cell infiltrates are variable in extent but they are often quite scanty. They tend to be more prominent around vessels and in the perimysial connective tissue than deeper in the endomysial connective tissue. The inflammatory cells consist of an admixture of lymphocytes, plasma cells, and macrophages. The lymphocytes have been shown to contain a relatively large proportion of B cells.[11]

Microvascular alterations are prominent in dermatomyositis. In both the childhood and adult forms, ultrastructural examination will disclose undulating tubular arrays in the endothelial cells of occasional intramuscular capillaries (Fig. 3–14). These structures were originally described in kidney biopsy specimens from patients with lupus erythematosus. Subsequently they have been

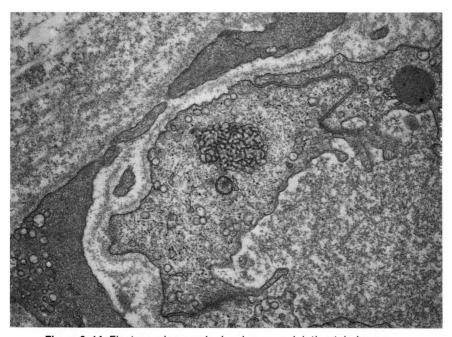

Figure 3-14. Electron micrograph showing an undulating tubular array within the cytoplasm of an endothelial cell. This muscle biopsy specimen was obtained from a 49-year-old woman with prominent perifascicular atrophy but minimal inflammatory cell infiltrates. ×37,500.

seen in association with a wide variety of connective tissue diseases, viral infections, and neoplasms.[22] In muscle specimens, however, they are highly characteristic of dermatomyositis. Similar alterations can be seen in specimens of skin. In the childhood form of dermatomyositis, there is a marked reduction in the number of capillaries per unit area (capillary density) within the areas of perifascicular atrophy. This loss of capillaries is difficult to demonstrate with routine frozen or paraffin-embedded sections but has been carefully documented by Carpenter et al.[30] from studies on epoxy-embedded sections. These authors attribute the distinctive perifascicular atrophy in these patients to progressive microvascular ischemia. Capillary necrosis and thrombosis also may be seen. Occasionally, larger vessels within the perimysium may be occluded (Fig. 3–15). Specimens from adults with dermatomyositis show undulating tubular arrays in endothelial cells but do not show a comparable reduction in the number of capillaries. Staining for alkaline phosphatase will show increased reactivity in capillaries and connective tissue in both adults and children.

Dermatomyositis in the adult has been associated with an increased risk of malignant neoplasms, especially in older men. The extent of this increased risk is controversial but is probably quite low.[1] Some studies have suggested that the increased risk, although small, also applies to women.[31] The morphologic features seen in adult dermatomyositis are the same whether or not the patient has an associated malignant neoplasm. No increased risk of neoplasia has been reported in children with dermatomyositis.

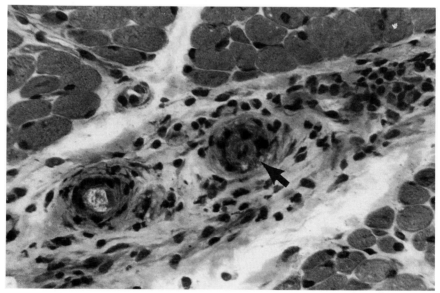

Figure 3-15. Occluded perimysial blood vessel *(arrow)* in a child with dermatomyositis. H&E, ×430.

Inclusion Body Myositis

Inclusion body myositis is being diagnosed with increasing frequency as more physicians become familiar with its clinical and histopathologic features. The condition was first delineated as a distinct entity by Yunis and Samaha[17] although earlier reports had described some of the light[32] and electron microscopic[16,18] features. Despite the relatively small number of reported cases, a rather characteristic set of clinical manifestations has emerged. Most of the patients have been middle-aged or elderly men with slowly progressive weakness. Women are apt to be affected at a somewhat younger age than men. Eisen et al.[33] have emphasized the bimodal age distribution among patients with this disease. Unlike most of the other inflammatory myopathies, distal weakness is often as marked as proximal weakness. Electrophysiologic studies often reveal apparent manifestations of neurogenic atrophy in addition to those of a myopathy. Serum muscle enzymes such as CK are variably elevated. Many of the patients follow a protracted course and generally are unresponsive to steroid therapy. Rarely, inclusion body myositis has been associated with other connective tissue–vascular diseases.[34,35]

The definitive diagnosis of this disorder can be made only by histopathologic study of muscle specimens. Muscle specimens from patients with inclusion body myositis show marked variation in myofiber size (Fig. 3–16). This variation is due to the presence of numerous moderately to markedly atrophic myofibers that are scattered individually and aggregated in small groups. In addition, some fibers may show moderate hypertrophy. Although the atrophy affects fibers of both types and resembles neurogenic atrophy, fiber type grouping indicative of reinnervation is not seen.

The most striking morphologic feature of this disease is the presence of irregular small vacuoles that are partially filled with fine granules. In frozen sections, the granules stain blue with H&E (Fig. 3–17) and reddish–purple with the modified trichrome technique. The vacuoles and their granular contents often show prominent esterase and acid phosphatase activity. Although these morphologic distinctive vacuoles are one of the most characteristic histologic features of inclusion body myositis, they are not pathognomonic of the disease and may be seen in a wide variety of other conditions.[36] Furthermore, the vacuoles are often inconspicuous in paraffin-embedded sections since the granular material is dissolved extensively during the tissue processing. By electron microscopy, the granules appear as loose or compact, membranous whorls (Fig. 3–18). Other myofibers may contain subsarcolemmal deposits of granular material that stain blue with H&E and reddish with the trichrome procedure. These deposits are further characterized by heavy staining with the NADH–TR and SDH reactions. Although these peripheral deposits may be partially vacuolated, they are actually abnormal deposits of mitochrondria as can be shown by electron microscopy. Some of the mitochrondria may display structural aberrations such as whorled cristae or intracristal paracrystalline arrays.

Scattered necrotic myofibers undergoing myophagocytosis and occasional

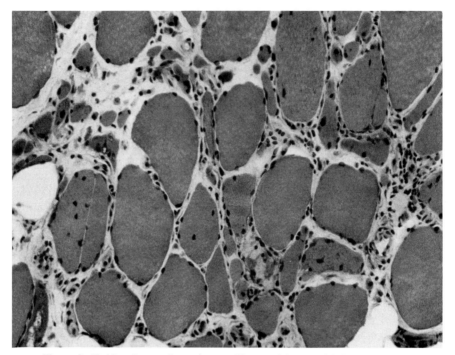

Figure 3-16. Muscle specimen from a 59-year-old man with inclusion body myositis. Note the marked variation in myofiber size, increased endomysial connective tissue, and moderately severe inflammatory cell infiltrates. H&E, ×175.

regenerating myofibers may be encountered. In addition, nonspecific degenerative changes such as cytoplasmic bodies may be present. The most significant alteration, however, is not readily detected by light microscopy. This is the presence of randomly oriented, fuzzy-appearing filaments. These filaments measure 15 to 18 nm in diameter and are of undetermined length. At higher magnification, some of the filaments appear to be tubular. They are found most commonly in the vicinity of the vacuoles and membranous whorls (Fig. 3–18). Sometimes, masses of filaments of a similar size and appearance may be encountered in myofiber nuclei (Fig. 3–19). Nuclei containing these filamentous inclusions are very rarely detected by light microscopy. When seen, the nuclei appear slightly enlarged and contain a homogeneous eosinophilic inclusion surrounded by marginated chromatin (Fig. 3–20). They must be distinguished from the large vesicular nuclei with prominent nucleoli, that are readily found in regenerating myofibers.

The nature of the abnormal intracytoplasmic and intranuclear filamentous material found in inclusion body myositis is unclear. When originally observed, Chou[16] suggested that the filaments may be myxovirus nucleocapsids. However, the filaments are straighter than most myxovirus filaments and, to date,

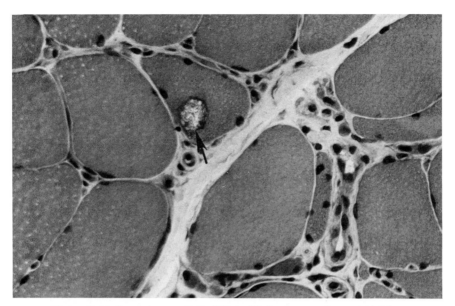

Figure 3-17. Vacuoles, partially filled with finely granular material *(arrow)*, are one of the features of inclusion body myositis. H&E, ×440.

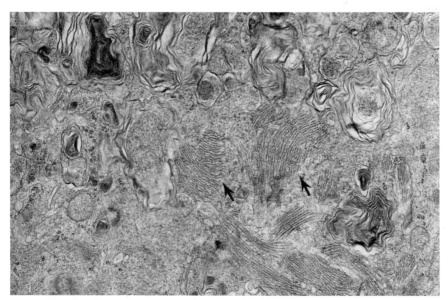

Figure 3-18. Electron micrograph showing roughly concentric osmiophilic lamella *(top)* that correspond to the granular vacuolar contents and skeins of the characteristic fuzzy-appearing filaments *(arrows)*. ×22,500.

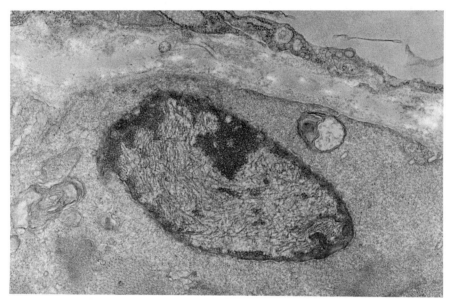

Figure 3-19. Electron micrograph showing additional fuzzy-appearing filaments within a myofiber nucleus. ×28,750.

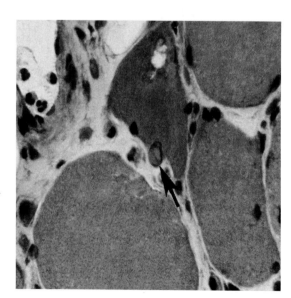

Figure 3-20. Rarely, nuclei that contain ill-defined eosinophilic inclusions *(arrow)* can be seen by light microscopy in specimens from patients with inclusion body myositis. A vacuole is also present in the same myofiber. H&E, ×440.

this virus has not been isolated. An adenovirus has been isolated from a muscle biopsy specimen from a patient with inclusion body myositis,[20] however, the significance of this finding remains to be determined. Yunis and Samaha[17] have emphasized the morphologic similarity to myosin filaments. Possibly, normal contractile proteins are altered by viral infection or immunologic injury to produce these characteristic structures. The ultrastructural demonstration of these abnormal filaments is essential for the definitive diagnosis of inclusion body myositis.

The endomysial connective tissue is often very unevenly increased, with the areas of maximal fibrosis found amoung the atrophic angular myofibers. These are often the same areas in which inflammatory cell infiltrates are most conspicuous. The inflammatory cells have been shown to contain a large proportion of T cells.[11] Quantitative studies by Carpenter et al.[19] have demonstrated an increased capillary density in this disorder. Rarely, undulating tubular arrays have been demonstrated in the capillary endothelial cells.[34]

Myositis and Other Connective Tissue Disorders

Idiopathic inflammatory myopathies, especially polymyositis and dermatomyositis, are commonly classified among the connective tissue disorders because of their presumed immunologic pathogenesis and their association with other disorders in this group of diseases. Some authors[1,4,28] classify these cases with clinically mixed diseases in a separate category. As many as 20 percent of patients with idiopathic inflammatory myopathy have concurrent connective tissue disorders, or develop subsequent evidence of them. The association seems especially prevalent with scleroderma (progressive systemic sclerosis). As many as 40 percent of patients with scleroderma have been found to have morphologic evidence of myositis.[4] In some of these patients, the morphologic changes were sufficiently similar to dermatomyositis to warrant using the term "sclerodermatomyositis." Arahata and Engel[11] have, however, reported a lower proportion of B cells in scleroderma than in dermatomyositis. Usually there is prominent proliferation of perimysial connective tissue and thickening of perimysial blood vessels. Nonspecific myopathic changes also may be seen. Localized scleroderma or morphea also may be accompanied by focal myofiber atrophy and inflammation.[37]

Five to 10 percent of patients with lupus erythematosus have been reported to have evidence of an inflammatory myopathy.[38] The histopathologic changes are similar to other cases of polymyositis and dermatomyositis. Prominent vacuolated fibers have been observed by several authors but these are more likely related to the therapeutic use of chloroquine.[39] Other patients have shown type II myofiber atrophy that can be attributed in part to the therapeutic use of corticosteroids.

Patients with rheumatoid disease often show a wide variety of histopathologic changes in muscle. The more severe cases will often show inflammatory cell infiltrates, myofiber atrophy including preferential type I myofiber atrophy, and nonspecific alterations such as targetoid fibers and ring fibers. In some patients, the inflammatory cell infiltrates will be localized and can be designated as interstitial myositis. Some of the milder cases show preferential atrophy of type IIB myofibers.[40] This may, in part, be due to disuse or therapeutic use of corticosteroids. More recently, cases of florid polymyositis have been reported in patients with rheumatoid arthritis who have been treated with penicillamine.[41]

Rarely, patients with Sjögren's syndrome may develop myositis.[34,35,42] The myositis may resemble polymyositis or dermatomyositis, including the presence of undulating tubular arrays within capillary endothelial cells. In some patients, the inflammatory cell infiltrates may contain a remarkably high proportion of plasma cells. Rarely, inclusion body myositis has been reported in association with Sjögren's syndrome.[34,35]

Eosinophilic fasciitis is a relatively recently described connective tissue disease characterized by peripheral eosinophilia and clinical manifestations that resemble scleroderma.[43,44] Histopathologic studies have shown normal skin, mild inflammation of the subcutaneous tissues, and prominent fibrosis and inflammation of the epimysium. Perivascular inflammatory cell infiltrates may be prominent. The inflammatory cells consist of eosinophils along with mononuclear cells. The underlying muscle generally shows only minimal inflammation and necrosis. The histopathologic alterations, including the characteristic distribution of the inflammatory cell infiltrates, are better seen in paraffin-embedded sections than frozen sections. Optimally, the specimen should include skin, subcutaneous tissue, and muscle in continuity.

Prominent histopathologic changes are seen in muscle from patients with polyarteritis; however, the major changes are those of the vasculitis. Small arteries may show intense inflammation and foci of fibrinoid necrosis (Fig. 3–21). The inflammatory cell infiltrate in the vessel wall includes polymorphonuclear leukocytes, eosinophils, and mononuclear cells. The fibrinoid necrosis and eosinophils are more difficult to identify in frozen sections than in paraffin-embedded sections. Muscle in the immediate vicinity of the necrotic vessels may contain mild inflammatory cell infiltrates. These include occasional eosinophils and plasma cells as well as more numerous lymphocytes and macrophages. In areas, the muscle fibers may be atrophic. In part this is due to neurogenic atrophy from involvement of peripheral nerves by the necrotizing vasculitis (see discussion under vasculitic neuropathies). In addition, the muscle may show type II myofiber atrophy. This is a nonspecific manifestation of the disease and a result of corticosteroid therapy. In other areas, the vasculitis may result in small infarcts. These lesions are characterized by groups of necrotic fibers including some that are vacuolated. The necrotic fibers are abnormally stained, granular, and devoid of cellular detail. Inflammatory cells are largely confined to the periphery of the infarcts and include intact and degenerating polymorphonuclear leukocytes. Other forms of vasculitis may be characterized by granulomatous involvement of the intramuscular vessel walls, again with minimal involvement of the muscle per se (Fig. 3–22).

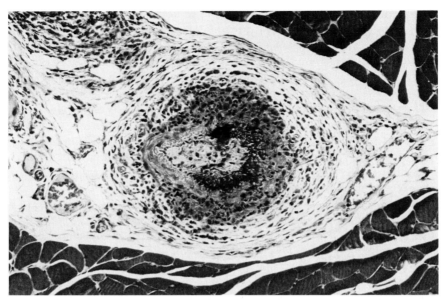

Figure 3-21. Paraffin-embedded muscle specimen showing typical changes of polyarteritis. Trichrome, × 220.

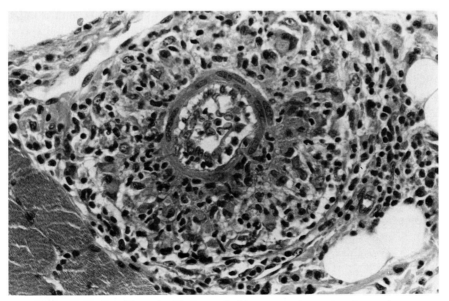

Figure 3-22. Paraffin-embedded muscle biopsy specimen showing a granulomatous vasculitis with minimal alterations in the surrounding myofibers. H&E, × 440.

Other Inflammatory Myopathies

Focal myositis is an inflammatory pseudotumor of skeletal muscle.[45] The lesions characteristically develop rapidly over a period of weeks and are found most often on the extremities. There is no clinical or laboratory evidence of a systemic disease. The lesions are circumscribed but poorly demarcated from the surrounding muscle. Histologically, the lesions display muscle fiber necrosis, regeneration, myofiber hypertrophy, lymphocytic infiltration, and interstitial fibrosis. In some patients there is also evidence of denervation. It has been suggested that denervation may play a role in the pathogenesis of these lesions. Rarely is there any history of local trauma. This lesion can be distinguished by the persistently normal ESR and normal CK levels from the unusual cases of polymyositis that begin as a focal lesion.[46]

Eosinophilic polymyositis[47] is a subacute inflammatory myopathy that is a component of the so-called "hypereosinophilic syndrome." This systemic illness is characterized by eosinophilia, anemia, hypergammaglobulinemia, edema, pulmonary infiltrates, cardiac involvement, livedo reticularis, Raynaud's phenomenon, subungual petechiae, peripheral neuropathy, and encephalopathy. Muscle involvement has been documented in a small number of patients and consists of myofiber degeneration, regeneration, and inflammation. The inflammatory cell infiltrates are composed predominantly of eosinophils. The inflammatory cells are found both in the interstitial tissues and about blood vessels. This process has also been reported in the form of a localized pseudotumor.[48]

Skeletal muscles commonly harbor granulomas in patients with sarcoidosis.[49] The granulomas are generally small and multiple although they may occasionally form a palpable mass. Some patients with sarcoidosis have clinical manifestations of a diffuse myopathy with proximal muscle weakness and atrophy. Histologically, the typical lesions are small noncaseating granulomas. They are composed of epithelioid cells and giant cells with an admixture of lymphocytes, plasma cells, and rare polymorphonuclear leukocytes. The granulomas (Fig. 3–23) are found predominantly in the perimysial connective tissue and about blood vessels. The surrounding muscle may show atrophy, especially of type II myofibers. Whether the granulomas are ever confined to muscle remains controversial. In at least some patients, granulomatous lesions were apparently limited to skeletal muscle and were accompanied by skin lesions that resembled dermatomyositis.[50] A granulomatous myositis that morphologically resembles sarcoid has been described in association with giant cell myocarditis and thymoma.[51]

Various parasites may involve skeletal muscle and produce inflammatory myopathies. One of the most commonly encountered parasites in skeletal muscle is Trichinella. Human infection results most often from the consumption of inadequately cooked pork. Larvae are released in the stomach and penetrate the walls of the duodenum and jejunum where they mature. The adults produce larvae that enter the systemic circulation and spread throughout the body. Muscle fibers of both types are parasitized by larvae that undergo further ma-

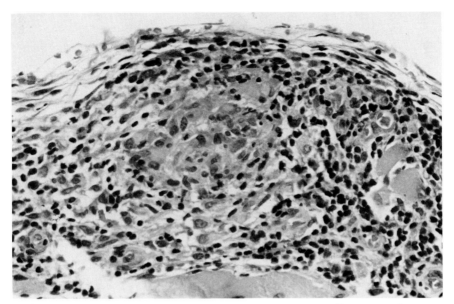

Figure 3-23. Paraffin-embedded section containing a small noncaseating granuloma from a woman with systemic sarcoidosis. H&E, ×500.

turation. During early stages, the coiled larva may be found within the interior of the myofibers.[52] After about 3 months, the enlarged larvae become surrounded by a collagenous capsule. Although the encysted larvae may remain viable for many years, calcification begins after 6 to 9 months (Fig. 3-24). The adjacent myofibers show a wide variety of nonspecific inflammatory and degenerative changes.

Toxoplasma cysts may be encountered in muscle specimens without evidence of an accompanying inflammatory reaction. Many of the other parasites that are known to affect skeletal muscle pose few diagnostic problems and will not be covered here.

Viruses are being identified with increasing frequency in cases of acute or subacute myositis.[3,14,23,53,54] In many of these patients, the virus has been one of the influenzal agents. The resulting diseases have ranged from mild myalgias to severe rhabdomyolysis and myoglobinuria.[23] Histologic studies in the more severe cases have shown myofiber necrosis and regeneration accompanied by inflammatory cell infiltrates. In some patients, undulating tubular arrays have been demonstrated within capillary endothelial cells.[23]

Although bacterial infections or superinfections (so-called tropical myositis) are an important cause of inflammatory muscle disease in many parts of the world, they are rarely seen in the United States. Tropical myositis is due to *Staphylococcus aureus* infections and involves especially the biceps, pectoral, gluteal, and quadriceps muscles in children and young adults. More recently, acute bacterial myositis due to *Vibrio vulnificus* has been described in individ-

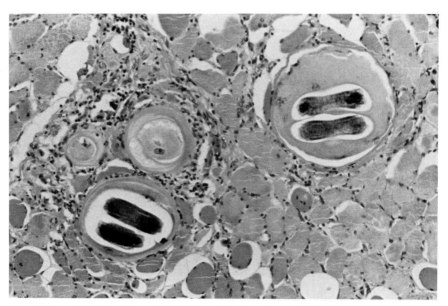

Figure 3-24. Paraffin-embedded section showing calcified encysted larvae of Trichinella. This was an incidental finding at autopsy. H&E, ×170.

uals who have wounds that become contaminated with seawater, or who have bacteremia from the consumption of seafood.[55] The illness is fulminating and leads to hypotension and leukopenia. Secondary necrotic lesions develop on the extremities. Histologic examination of these lesions has shown necrosis of skin, subcutaneous tissue, and underlying skeletal muscle. Necrosis of the blood vessels results in extensive hemorrhage as well as inflammation. Since the organism is common in marine environments, infections with this agent may be more frequent than currently recognized.

Factitious Myositis
It is important for the pathologist to consider the possibility of factitious myositis whenever unexpected inflammatory reactions are encountered in muscle specimens. Specimens removed inadvertently from sites subjected to previous electromyographic needle examinations, injections, and surgical procedures will show varying degrees of myofiber necrosis, regeneration, and fibrosis (Fig. 3-25). Occasionally, a needle tract can be identified by a linear band of necrosis or a strand of collagenous tissue oriented perpendicular to the long axis of the muscle. Less commonly, prior injections may result in the formation of non-caseating granulomas. This has been documented following intramuscular diphtheria, pertussis, tetanus (DPT) injections.[56] The granulomas contained epithelioid cells, lymphocytes, and plasma cells but no giant cells or organisms. Histiocytes contained granular material that stained blue with H&E and red with the PAS technique. The presence of aluminum, used in the preparation

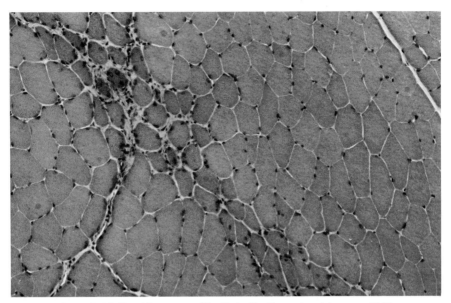

Figure 3-25. Factitious myositis. Note the linear tract from an EMG needle. H&E, ×175.

of the vaccine, was demonstrated by an acid-stable green fluorescence following staining with morin.

References

1. Bohan A, Peter JB: Polymyositis and dermatomyositis. N Engl J Med 292:344–347, 1975; 292:403–407, 1975.
2. Whitaker JN: Inflammatory myopathy: A review of etiologic and pathogenetic factors. Muscle Nerve 5:573–592, 1982.
3. Mastaglia FL, Ojeda VJ: Inflammatory myopathies: Part I. Ann Neurol 17:215–227, 1985; 17:317–323, 1985.
4. Currie S: Inflammatory myopathies. Part I: Polymyositis and related disorders. In Walton JN (ed): Disorders of Voluntary Muscle, 4th ed. Edinburgh, Churchill Livingstone, 1981, pp 525–568.
5. Carpenter S, Karpati G: The major inflammatory myopathies of unknown cause. Pathol Annu 16 (Part 2):205–237, 1981.
6. Kakulas BA: Observations on the etiology of polymyositis. In Pearson CM, Mostofi FK (eds): The Striated Muscle. Baltimore, Williams & Wilkins, 1973, pp 485–497.
7. Whitaker JN, Engel WK: Vascular deposits of immunoglobulin and complement in idiopathic inflammatory myopathy. N Engl J Med 286:333–338, 1972.
8. Heffner RR, Barron SA, Jenis EH, Valeski JE: Skeletal muscle in polymyositis. Immunohistochemical study. Arch Pathol Lab Med 103:310–313, 1979.
9. Pachman LM, Cooke N: Juvenile dermatomyositis. A clinical and immunologic study. J Pediatr 96:226–234, 1980.

10. Venables PJW, Mumford PA, Maini RN: Antibodies to nuclear antigens in polymyositis: Relationship to autoimmune overlap syndromes and carcinoma. Ann Rheum Dis 40:217–223, 1981.
11. Arahata K, Engel AG: Monoclonal antibody analysis of mononuclear cells in myopathies. I. Quantitation of subsets according to diagnosis and sites of accumulation and demonstration and counts of muscle fibers invaded by T cells. Ann Neurol 16:193–208, 1984.
12. Chou SM, Gutmann L: Picornavirus-like crystals in subacute polymyositis. Neurology 20:205–213, 1970.
13. Mastaglia FL, Walton JN: Coxsackie virus-like particles in skeletal muscle from a case of polymyositis. J Neurol Sci 11:593–599, 1970.
14. Tang TT, Sedmak GV, Siegsmund KA, McCreadie SR: Chronic myopathy associated with Coxsackie virus type A9: A combined electron microscopical and viral isolation study. N Engl J Med 292:608–611, 1975.
15. Katsuragi S, Miyayama MD, Takeuchi T: Picornavirus-like inclusions in polymyositis—aggregation of glycogen particles of the same size. Neurology 31:1476–1480, 1981.
16. Chou SM: Myxovirus-like structures and accompanying nuclear changes in chronic polymyositis. Arch Pathol 86:649–658, 1968.
17. Yunis EJ, Samaha FJ: Inclusion body myositis. Lab Invest 25:240–248, 1971.
18. Sato T, Walker DL, Peters HA, et al.: Chronic polymyositis and myxovirus-like inclusions. Arch Neurol 24:409–418, 1971.
19. Carpenter S, Karpati G, Heller I, Eisen A: Inclusion body myositis: A distinct variety of idiopathic inflammatory myopathy. Neurology 28:8–17, 1978.
20. Mikol J, Felten-Papaiconomou A, Ferchal F, et al.: Inclusion-body myositis: Clinicopathological studies and isolation of an adenovirus type 2 from muscle biopsy specimen. Ann Neurol 11:576–581, 1982.
21. Carpenter S, Karpati G, Rothman S, Watters G: The childhood type of dermatomyositis. Neurology 26:952–962, 1976.
22. Grimley PM, Schaff Z: Significance of tubuloreticular inclusions in the pathobiology of human diseases. Pathobiol Annu 6:221–257, 1976.
23. Gamboa ET, Eastwood AB, Hays AP, et al.: Isolation of influenza virus from muscle in myoglobinuric polymyositis. Neurology 29:1323–1335, 1979.
24. MacDonald RD, Engel AG: The cytoplasmic body: Another structural anomaly of the Z disk. Acta Neuropathol 14:99–107, 1969.
25. Schochet SS Jr, McCormick WF: Polymyositis with intranuclear inclusions. Arch Neurol 28:280–283, 1973.
26. Engel AG, Arahata K: Monoclonal antibody analysis of mononuclear cells in myopathies. II. Phenotypes of autoinvasive cells in polymyositis and inclusion body myositis. Ann Neurol 16:209–215, 1984.
27. Jerusalem F: Circulatory disorders and pathology of intramuscular blood vessels. In Mastaglia FL, Walton JN (eds): Skeletal Muscle Pathology. Edinburgh, Churchill Livingstone, 1982, pp 537–560.
28. DeVere R, Bradley WG: Polymyositis: Its presentation, morbidity and mortality. Brain 98:637–666, 1975.
29. Banker BQ: Dermatomyositis of childhood. Ultrastructural alterations of muscle and intramuscular blood vessels. J Neuropathol Exp Neurol 34:46–75, 1975.
30. Carpenter S, Karpati G, Rothman S, Watters G: The childhood type of dermatomyositis. Neurology 26:952–962, 1976.
31. Barnes BE: Dermatomyositis and malignancy: A review of the literature. Ann Intern Med 84:68–76, 1976.

32. Adams RD, Kakulas BA, Samaha FJ: A myopathy with cellular inclusions. Trans Am Neurol Assoc 90:213–216, 1965.
33. Eisen A, Berry K, Gibson G: Inclusion body myositis (IBM): Myopathy or neuropathy? Neurology 33:1109–1114, 1983.
34. Chad D, Good P, Adelman L, et al.: Inclusion body myositis associated with Sjögren's syndrome. Arch Neurol 39:186–188, 1982.
35. Gutmann L, Govindan S, Riggs JE, Schochet SS Jr: Inclusion body myositis and Sjögren's syndrome. Arch Neurol 42:1021–1022, 1985.
36. Fukuhara N, Kumamoto T, Tsubaki T: Rimmed vacuoles. Acta Neuropathol 51:229–236, 1980.
37. Miike T, Ohtani Y, Hattori S, et al.: Childhood-type myositis and linear scleroderma. Neurology 33:928–930, 1983.
38. Foote RA, Kimbrough SM, Stevens JC: Lupus myositis. Muscle Nerve 5:65–68, 1982.
39. Itabashi HH, Kokmen E: Chloroquine neuromyopathy. A reversible granulovacuolar myopathy. Arch Pathol 93:209–218, 1972.
40. Brooke MH, Kaplan H: Muscle pathology in rheumatoid arthritis, polymyalgia rheumatica, and polymyositis. A histochemical study. Arch Pathol 94:101–118, 1972.
41. Morgan GJ Jr, McGuire JL, Ochoa J: Penicillamine-induced myositis in rheumatoid arthritis. Muscle Nerve 4:137–140, 1981.
42. Ringel SP, Forstot JZ, Tan EM, et al.: Sjögren's syndrome and polymyositis or dermatomyositis. Arch Neurol 39:157–163, 1982.
43. Barnes L, Rodman GP, Medsger TA Jr, Short D: Eosinophilic fasciitis. A pathologic study of twenty cases. Am J Pathol 96:493–518, 1979.
44. Simon DB, Ringel SP, Sufit RL: Clinical spectrum of fascial inflammation. Muscle Nerve 5:525–537, 1982.
45. Heffner RR, Barron SA: Denervating changes in focal myositis, a benign inflammatory pseudotumor. Arch Pathol Lab Med 104:261–264, 1980.
46. Heffner RR, Barron SA: Polymyositis beginning as a focal process. Arch Neurol 38:339–442, 1981.
47. Layzer RB, Shearn MA, Satya-Murti S: Eosinophilic polymyositis. Ann Neurol 1:65–71, 1977.
48. Agrawai BL, Giesen PC: Eosinophilic myositis: An unusual cause of pseudotumor and eosinophilia. JAMA 246:7071, 1981.
49. Gardner-Thorpe C: Muscle weakness due to sarcoid myopathy. Six case reports and an evaluation of steroid therapy. Neurology 22:917–928, 1972.
50. Itoh J, Akiguchi I, Midorikawa R, Kameyama M: Sarcoid myopathy with typical rash of dermatomyositis. Neurology 30:1118–1121, 1980.
51. Namba T, Bruknner NG, Grob D: Idiopathic giant cell polymyositis. Arch Neurol 31:27–30, 1974.
52. Gross B, Ochoa J: Trichinosis: Clinical report and histochemistry of muscle. Muscle Nerve 2:394–398, 1979.
53. Congy F, Hauw JJ, Wang A, Moulias R: Influenzal acute myositis in the elderly. Neurology 30:877–878, 1980.
54. Ruff RL, Secrist D: Viral studies in benign acute childhood myositis. Arch Neurol 39:261–263, 1982.
55. Kelly MT, McCormick WF: Acute bacterial myositis caused by Vibrio vulnificus. JAMA 246:72–73, 1981.
56. Mrak RE: Muscle granulomas following intramuscular injection. Muscle Nerve 5:637–639, 1982.

chapter 4

Dystrophies

The muscular dystrophies are an ill-defined group of progressive, degenerative myopathies. They are genetically determined but despite extensive investigation, their etiology and pathogenesis remain unknown. The diseases included among the dystrophies are arbitrarily limited by conventional usage. A number of myopathies, to which these general statements would apply, are not customarily regarded as muscular dystrophies. Such is the case with some of the so-called metabolic myopathies such as the mitochondrial myopathies. Other myopathies have been removed from the "dystrophies" as our knowledge of their pathogenesis has evolved. For example, some patients formerly considered to have limb girdle dystrophy are now known to have adult-onset acid maltase deficiency, an incompletely elucidated disorder of carbohydrate metabolism.

DUCHENNE MUSCULAR DYSTROPHY

Duchenne muscular dystrophy is the most pernicious of the disorders classified among the muscular dystrophies. This disease is inherited as an X-linked recessive trait but there is a high rate of spontaneous mutations. Duchenne muscular dystrophy is variously estimated to have an incidence of 13 to 33/100,000 newborn males and a prevalence of 4 to 7/100,000 males. Of these cases, nearly one third are thought to be the result of new mutations.[1] All affected males show the full expression of the disease. Rarely, the disease may be manifested in phenotypic females who have Turner syndrome or mosaicism of the X chromosomes. Occasionally, female carriers may be mildly symptomatic. Rarely, they have been reported to show severe, progressive disease as the result of incomplete lyonization of the X chromosome.[2,3]

Although the disease clearly begins in utero, the earliest recognized symptoms are generally delayed walking, clumsiness, and frequent falls. The manifestations of the disease are often detected earlier by parents who previously have had an affected son. The disease is relentlessly progressive although periods of rapid growth and development may lead to the spurious impression of transient improvement. Weakness usually begins in the pelvic musculature and spreads to the pectoral girdle and proximal muscles of the upper limbs. So-called "pseudohypertrophy," enlargement due to adipose replacement, is seen commonly in the calves.

Most patients lose their ability to walk between the ages of 7 and 12 years. Intercurrent illnesses, treated with enforced bed rest, often accelerate loss of ambulation. Contractures and scoliosis become more pronounced after the patients are confined to wheelchairs. The skeletal deformities and rarefaction of bone can be attributed to the muscular weakness and disuse. Mild mental retardation is common. The pathogenesis of this aspect of the disease is unclear. It is considered to be more severe than can be explained by the physical handicap alone.[4] However, no consistent morphologic abnormalities have been observed in the nervous system.

The patients eventually become bedridden and most die by the beginning of the third decade. Survival beyond the age of 25 years is very rare. Death is usually the result of intercurrent infection, respiratory failure, or cardiac failure. Cardiac involvement is common among patients with Duchenne dystrophy and occasionally occurs in female carriers.[5] It is usually manifested by electrocardiographic abnormalities or even arrhythmias. Chronic myocardial failure is uncommon. Morphologic studies generally have shown interstitial fibrosis that may be most severe in the posterobasal portion of the left ventricular wall.

Duchenne muscular dystrophy is characterized by marked increase in the serum CK level. The elevation is most prominent early in childhood when it may be 100 to 300 times greater than normal. Elevated CK levels may be demonstrated long before other clinical manifestations of the disease appear. For this reason, several authors recommend the determination of CK levels in all male infants with any type of developmental delay.[6] Prenatal assay of CK activity in fetal blood had been reported to identify some male fetuses with Duchenne dystrophy,[7] however, further studies have shown that this procedure may be unreliable.[8] In older patients, in the later stages of the disease, the enzyme activity may be only one to five times greater than normal.

Histopathology

Muscle biopsy specimens from patients with Duchenne muscular dystrophy show a wide spectrum of histopathologic abnormalities. None alone is specific for the disorder and the relative prominence of the various abnormalities changes during the course of the disease.

In almost all patients, there is increased variation in myofiber size (Figs. 4–1 and 4–2). This may be mild in specimens from very young patients but becomes more prominent with progression of the disease. The variation in myofiber size is due to the presence of both hypertrophied and atrophic myofibers. Both major fiber types are affected. However, virtually none of the small myofibers are as angular as the atrophic myofibers in neurogenic disease. The hypertrophied myofibers generally have rounded contours when seen in cross-

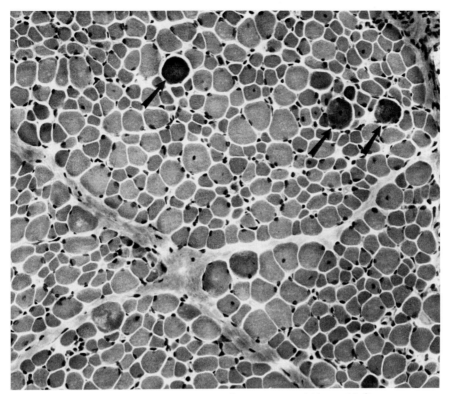

Figure 4-1. Muscle biopsy specimen from a 1-year-old boy with Duchenne muscular dystrophy. This clinically asymptomatic child was found to have a markedly elevated CK level while hospitalized for a febrile illness. The specimen shows prominently increased variation in myofiber sizes due to the presence of hypertrophied and atrophic myofibers. Note also the dark-staining opaque fibers *(arrows)*. H&E, ×200.

section. In the younger patients with actively progressive disease, at least some of the large fibers stain excessively dark with almost all of the staining techniques used on frozen or paraffin-embedded sections. These large, dark-stained fibers are called *hyalinized* or *opaque fibers* (Figs. 4-1 and 4-3). Many workers regard them to be the result of hypercontraction in myofibers undergoing segmental necrosis above or below the plane of the section being examined. Although they are found in virtually all cases of Duchenne muscular dystrophy, they are not pathognomonic of this disease. Occasional opaque fibers can be seen in other muscle disorders and even in otherwise normal skeletal muscle that has been processed suboptimally. In Duchenne muscular dystrophy, the opaque fibers have been shown histochemically to contain excess calcium.[9] The increased calcium content may be responsible for the overly contracted state of the opaque fibers. The abnormal ingress of this ion may occur through

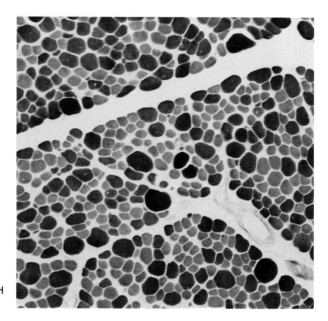

Figure 4-2. The variation in myofiber sizes involves fibers of both major types. ATPase, pH 9.4, ×200.

membrane defects in otherwise intact myofibers. Mokri and Engel[10] have demonstrated by light and electron microscopy, focal, wedge-shaped lesions in the periphery of nonnecrotic myofibers in patients with Duchenne muscular dystrophy. Within the lesions, myofilaments were sparse, sarcotubular profiles were dilated, and there was abnormal permeability to peroxidase. Mokri and Engel have proposed that these delta-shaped defects constitute the fundamental lesion

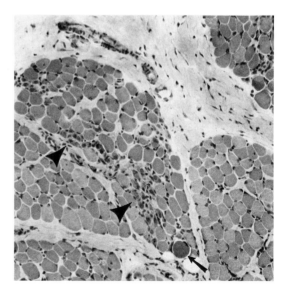

Figure 4-3. Degenerating and regenerating myofibers are typically found in small clusters *(arrowheads)*. Note also the hyalinized opaque fiber *(arrow)*. H&E, ×410.

in the cytopathology of Duchenne muscular dystrophy. The delta lesions have been demonstrated in preclinical and early cases of Duchenne muscular dystrophy.[11] Carpenter and Karpati[12] have suggested that focal lysis of the plasma membrane is the initial morphologic lesion since this alteration was always seen in necrotic fibers and only occasionally seen in nonnecrotic fibers. Although they regarded the influx of calcium to be involved in the production of the myofiber necrosis, they did not consider the hypercontraction as a step in its evolution. Schmalbruch[13] described focal loss of the plasma membrane as an antecedent to myofiber necrosis regardless of the disease in which it occurred. While these ultrastructural studies have added to our understanding of the pathogenesis of the disease, electron microscopy has a very limited role in the diagnosis of Duchenne muscular dystrophy.

Some muscle specimens from patients with Duchenne muscular dystrophy show a relatively high proportion of type I myofibers. Dubowitz and Brooke[14] have described deficiency of type IIB myofibers and the presence of numerous type IIC fibers in some of their cases. Generally we have found no significant alterations in the proportions or distribution of the major fiber types (see Fig. 4–2).

Probably the diagnostically most significant lesion is the presence of small clusters of degenerating and regenerating myofibers (Figs. 4–3 and 4–4). The degenerating myofibers display varying stages of necrosis and may appear hyalinized, liquefied, or abnormally granular. Eventually the necrotic myofibers undergo myophagocytosis (Fig. 4–5). Nonnecrotic degenerative changes such as vacuolation, ring fibers, and whorled fibers are inconspicuous. The regenerating myofibers are relatively small and have amphophilic cytoplasm. The characteristic amphophilic (reddish–blue) color of the regenerating myofibers is more readily seen in frozen than in paraffin-embedded sections. The regenerating myofibers have large vesicular nuclei that are often located in the interior of the fibers. Although ultimately regenerative activity may be insufficient to compensate for the degeneration, abundant regenerating myofibers are a characteristic feature of specimens obtained early in the course of this disease.[15] A variable number of mononuclear inflammatory cells, predominantly macrophages, are found within the endomysial connective tissue among the degenerating and regenerating myofibers (see Fig. 4–5). The degenerating fibers undergoing myophagocytosis and the accompanying cellular infiltrates can be preferentially stained with the nonspecific esterase reaction while the regenerating myofibers can be selectively stained with the alkaline phosphatase technique. In contrast to many inflammatory myopathies, the connective tissue does not show enhanced staining with the alkaline phosphatase technique. Some authors have advocated the use of the latter staining reaction to facilitate distinction between these two categories of disease. We have not found the alkaline phosphatase procedure sufficiently reliable for this purpose.

Another important histopathologic feature of Duchenne muscular dystrophy is progressive endomysial fibrosis. Early in the course of the illness, there is only a mild increase of fibrous tissue that is largely confined to the foci of

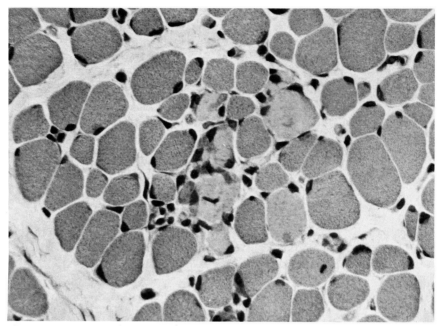

Figure 4-4. During the early stages of degeneration the necrotic myofibers appear liquefied. H&E, ×410.

degeneration and regeneration. With progression of the disease, the fibrosis becomes more pronounced and widespread. The fibrosis may be less evident in frozen sections than paraffin-embedded sections where it is accentuated by artifactual shrinkage of the entrapped myofibers (Figs. 4-6 and 4-7). Although the epi- and perimysial connective tissues also appear more abundant, only the increase in the endomysial connective tissue should be regarded as diagnostically significant. In very advanced cases, there is prominent adipose replacement. Eventually, specimens will consist of abundant fibroadipose tissue with only rare remaining myofibers. Intrafusal fibers within muscle spindles are more resistant to the degenerative changes than the extrafusal fibers. In some specimens, persistent muscle spindles may be the only evidence that a mass of fibroadipose tissue was formerly muscle.

Blood vessels within muscle specimens from patients with Duchenne muscular dystrophy often show progressive mural sclerosis. This is more conspicuous in the larger vessels and in the more advanced cases. These changes are sufficiently prominent that some workers had suggested that vascular occlusion was of pathogenetic significance.[16] This has not been supported by more recent studies. A morphometric analysis of the muscle microvasculature by Jerusalem et al.[17] disclosed increased capillary size, a reduced number of pinocytotic vesicles, and reduplication of the basal lamina but no evidence of capillary occlusion. No significant alterations have been documented in the intramuscular

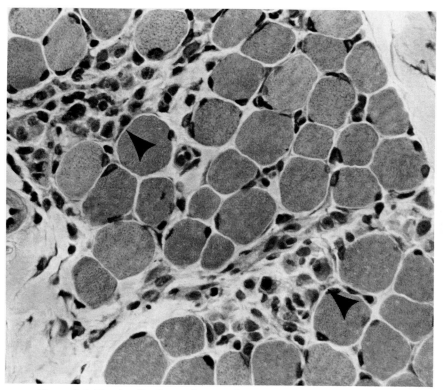

Figure 4-5. Focal collections of macrophages partially surrounded by basement membranes *(arrows)* indicate where necrotic fibers have undergone myophagocytosis. Note also the small number of interstitial mononuclear cells. H&E, ×410.

nerves. The neuromuscular junctions show degeneration of the postsynaptic folds and simplification of the postsynaptic regions similar to the changes seen in myasthenia gravis. However, these junctional alterations are not accompanied by a reduction in acetylcholine receptor or extrajunctional spread of the receptor.[18]

Although collectively these histopathologic changes are rather characteristic of Duchenne muscular dystrophy, this diagnosis should not be rendered without careful consideration of correlative clinical data.

Carrier Detection

Despite extensive investigations, which in more recent years have focused on membrane defects and imbalance between protein synthesis and degradation,[19,20] the pathogenesis of Duchenne muscular dystrophy remains unknown. Currently, Duchenne dystrophy is an incurable disease for which therapy is merely supportive. Therefore, genetic counseling is important in order to re-

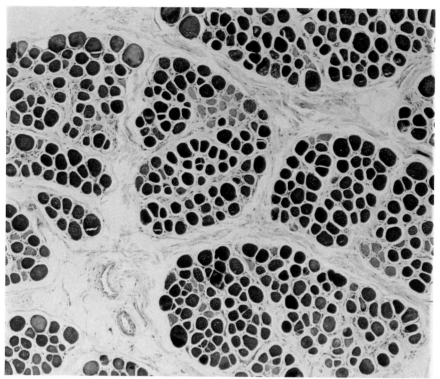

Figure 4-6. Paraffin-embedded muscle biopsy specimen from a 5-year-old boy with Duchenne muscular dystrophy. He was described as having big muscles but unable to keep up with his playmates. Note the increased endomysial connective tisue. Trichrome, ×80.

duce the incidence of additional affected patients. Because of the high rate of spontaneous mutations, this approach cannot be expected to eliminate the disease.

On the basis of careful clinical and laboratory studies, women at risk can be classified as definite, probable, and possible carriers. In part, this classification can be accomplished from pedigree analysis. Women with an affected son and a family history of other cases on the maternal side are regarded as definite carriers. Women with two or more affected sons but no family history of the disease are considered to be probable carriers. Women with a single affected son and no family history of the disease are classified as possible carriers. Since most carriers manifest at least some evidence of harboring the defective gene, many different clinical and laboratory studies have been employed in order to refine this categorization.[21]

At the present time, evaluation of serum muscle enzymes, especially CK, is the most widely used procedure. About 50 to 70 percent of definite carriers can be identified in this manner when multiple determinations are performed.[22]

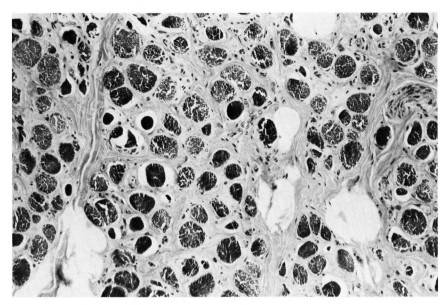

Figure 4-7. Paraffin-embedded specimen of psoas muscle obtained at the time of autopsy from a 17-year-old man with Duchenne muscular dystrophy. Trichrome, ×250.

The results, however, are influenced by seasonal variation, physical activity, the use of certain drugs, and may be spuriously low during pregnancy. There is evidence that more reliable data can be obtained if the serum enzyme determinations are performed during early childhood.

Other studies that have been advocated for carrier detection include electromyography, electrocardiography, determination of muscle protein synthesis, evaluation of membrane spectrin II phosphorylation, and evaluation of erythrocyte morphology. Histologic studies on muscle biopsy specimens may provide contributory information in the unusual carriers that are overtly symptomatic.[23] More often, however, muscle biopsy specimens from carriers show no abnormalities or merely minor nonspecific abnormalities that are difficult to interpret.

BECKER DYSTROPHY

This is a milder form of X-linked muscular dystrophy. It is about one tenth as common as Duchenne muscular dystrophy from which it is distinguished, clinically, by the later onset of symptoms and relatively slow progression.[23,24] There is considerable variation in severity among families with the disease, however, cases within a given family generally pursue a similar course.[25] Individuals affected with this disease usually do not become symptomatic until the latter half of the first or the second decades. Occasionally, the onset of symptoms has not been noted until the third decade. The initial manifestations are related to weakness of the pelvic girdle and proximal muscles of the lower limbs. Involvement of the shoulder girdle and upper limbs usually follows in a few years. Pseudohypertrophy of the calves is common. Skeletal deformities and contractures may occur but are less severe than in Duchenne dystrophy. A characteristic pes cavus deformity, originally noted by Becker, was observed in a large proportion of the patients reported by Ringel et al.[26] Cardiac involvement, manifested by electrocardiographic abnormalities, has been noted in at least some of the patients. The course of the disease is variable but generally is less pernicious than Duchenne muscular dystrophy. In the series reported by Bradley et al.,[25] the mean age for loss of ambulation was 35 years and some of their patients survived into the seventh decade. Ringel et al.[26] noted loss of ambulation at a somewhat earlier age in their cases. The serum CK levels are elevated but to a lesser degree than in Duchenne muscular dystrophy.

The histopathologic alterations encountered in these patients are varied. In some patients, the abnormalities have been described as being similar to those seen in Duchenne muscular dystrophy. More recent reports,[25,26] however, and the findings in our own patients, disclose as many differences as similarities. The muscle specimens show markedly increased variation in myofiber size (Figs. 4–8 and 4–9). This is due to the presence of hypertrophied myofibers and numerous moderately to markedly atrophic myofibers. Little or no type I myofiber predominance is seen. The large opaque myofibers, so characteristic of Duchenne muscular dystrophy, are few in number and are found in less than half of the muscle specimens. Necrotic myofibers undergoing myophagocytosis and basophilic regenerating myofibers are less numerous. Inflammatory cell infiltrates are rare. Endomysial fibrosis is present but highly variable in extent. Probably because of the protracted course of the disease, internalized nuclei and fiber splitting are conspicuous. Occasional fibers show structural abnormalities such as ring fibers, moth-eaten fibers, and whorled fibers. Internalized capillaries, i.e., capillaries that appear to be within otherwise intact myofibers, have been described in Becker dystrophy[27] but are not unique to this disorder (see Fig. 2–14). Ringel et al.[26] have described the histopathologic changes in Becker dystrophy as having features in common with both Duchenne dystrophy and limb girdle dystrophy. By contrast, Bradley et al.[25] described the histopathology of Becker dystrophy as having features of chronic myopathy and chronic neuropathy. Similar findings were reported by Goebel et al.[28] in biopsy specimens obtained from two of the patients originally reported clinically by Becker. One of the major differences among these reports is the interpretation of the pathogenesis of the small atrophic myofibers, i.e., whether they are merely the result of fiber splitting or whether they are the result of denervation. Group atrophy, pyknotic nuclear clumps, small angular myofibers, and even fiber-type grouping were described in a series of 14 cases of Becker dystrophy reported by ten Houten and De Visser.[29] As indicated by

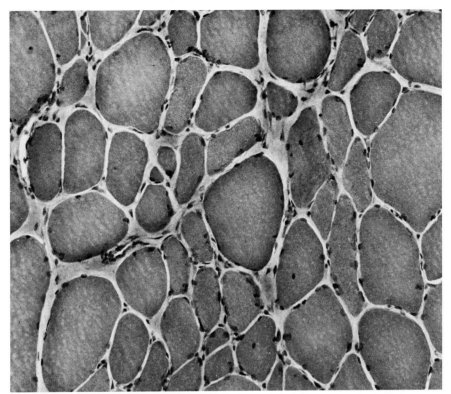

Figure 4-8. Muscle biopsy specimen from a 14-year-old boy with Becker muscular dystrophy. Note the presence of both hypertrophied myofibers and atrophic myofibers, along with a mild increase in the quantity of endomysial connective tissue. H&E, ×400.

these authors, neurogenic features are being reported with increasing frequency in this disease.

Although the morphologic findings in muscle specimens from these patients can substantiate a clinical diagnosis of Becker dystrophy, they are not by themselves diagnostic. The female carriers of this disorder may have elevated serum CK levels but are not symptomatic.

FACIOSCAPULOHUMERAL DYSTROPHY

Facioscapulohumeral dystrophy is probably a collection of disorders, a syndrome, rather than a single disease. The usual forms of the facioscapulohumeral syndrome are dominantly inherited. They are less common than Duchenne muscular dystrophy and have been estimated to have a prevalence of about two per million individuals.[1] Most are slowly progressive and do not

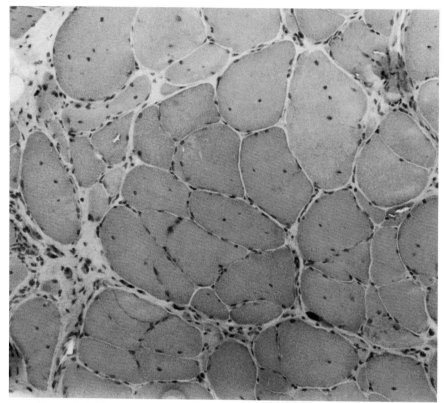

Figure 4-9. Muscle biopsy specimen from a man in his late twenties with Becker dystrophy. The patient had chronic proximal muscle weakness, marked hypertrophy of the calves, and myopathic changes by EMG. H&E, × 175. *(Slide provided by Dr. Hans Goebel, University of Maine.)*

significantly shorten life expectancy, but they are highly variable in their severity. The clinical manifestations usually become apparent during adolescence or early adult life and include slowly progressive weakness and atrophy of the facial muscles, shoulder girdle, and proximal limb muscles. In at least some of the patients, there is also involvement of the pelvic girdle and peroneal muscles. Weakness of the facial muscles is often the initial manifestation and results in pouting lips and a distinctive smile. The patients often sleep with their eyes partially open and are unable to drink with a straw or to whistle. The involvement of the shoulder girdle results in scapular winging, drooping shoulders, protruding clavicles, and accessory axillary creases. Characteristically, the deltoid muscles remain remarkably uninvolved both clinically and morphologically. This deltoid sparing is significant in both the clinical diagnosis and in the selection of muscle biopsy sites. Preservation of the bulk of the forearm in association with the atrophy of the upper arm results in a distinctive "Popeye" appearance. Pelvic and lower trunk weakness may result in lordosis while involvement of the peroneal muscles may result in a foot drop. Occasional patients have the peroneal weakness as their initial manifestation and only later develop weakness of the shoulder girdle. Some authors consider patients with this pattern of muscle involvement to have a different disease, scapuloperoneal dystrophy. However, the eventual development of facial weakness in about half of these individuals is regarded as evidence of a close relation to facioscapulohumeral dystrophy. Brooke[30] has described the occurrence of another variant of facioscapulohumeral dystrophy with initial manifestations becoming apparent during the first 2 years of life. This is a more pernicious form of the disease that rapidly leads to severe disability.

Morphologic studies on patients with facioscapulohumeral dystrophy disclose histopathologic alterations that are as varied as the clinical manifestations. In the less severely affected individuals, muscle specimens may show only increased variation in myofiber size (Fig. 4–10). This is due to the presence of occasional moderately hypertrophied myofibers and scattered atrophic myofibers. The atrophic myofibers may be rounded or angular-like denervated myofibers (Fig. 4–11). These may or may not stain darkly with the NADH–TR reaction. Other alterations that may be evident include whorled fibers, "motheaten" fibers, and lobulated fibers (Fig. 4–11). The lobulated fibers are usually best seen with the NADH–TR reaction (Fig. 4–12). These fibers also may be seen in limb girdle dystrophy.[31] Although not diagnostic, we have encountered them especially commonly in patients with facioscapulohumeral dystrophy. Rare necrotic myofibers, increased numbers of internal nuclei, and mildly increased endomysial fibrosis are also seen in many of these patients.

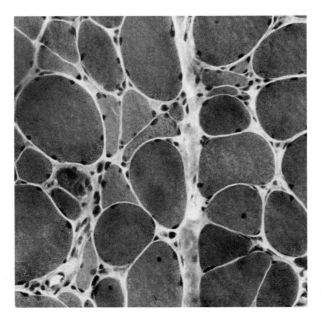

Figure 4-10. Muscle biopsy from a boy with facioscapulohumeral dystrophy. His mother and sister were similarly affected. Note the variation in myofiber size, with scattered angular atrophic myofibers and mildly increased endomysial connective tissue. Trichrome, × 330.

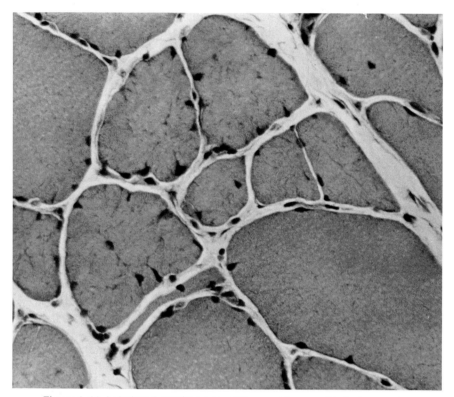

Figure 4-11. Lobulated myofibers in a 37-year-old man with facioscapulo-humeral dystrophy. The distinctive appearance of the lobulated myofibers results from disorganization of the intermyofibrillar network. H&E, ×410.

Some of the more severely affected individuals may have more prominent variation in myofiber size with marked hypertrophy of type II fibers. In addition, there may be conspicuous inflammatory cell infiltrates. Although these changes resemble inflammatory myopathy, they have been interpreted as a stage in the evolution of facioscapulohumeral dystrophy.[32,33] We have studied two patients with facioscapulohumeral dystrophy in whom the deltoid muscles were nearly normal while the supraspinatus muscles showed marked variation in myofiber size, inflammation, and severe interstitial fibrosis (Fig. 4-13).

These various forms of the facioscapulohumeral syndrome are considered to be dystrophies with myopathic changes on EMG and CK levels that are at least three or four times higher than normal. In addition, there are patients who have virtually identical clinical findings but show neurogenic alterations by EMG and on morphologic study of muscle specimens (Fig. 4-14). The precise relation between these cases of so-called "neurogenic facioscapulohumeral syndrome" and the spinal muscular atrophies remains to be elucidated.[29]

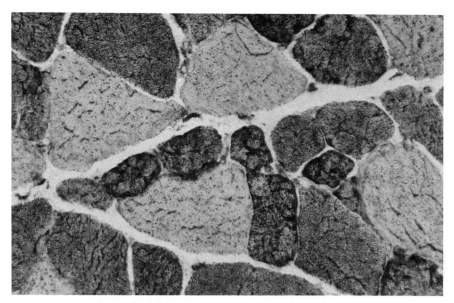

Figure 4-12. The lobulated fibers are often mildly atrophic type I myofibers. NADH–TR, ×40.

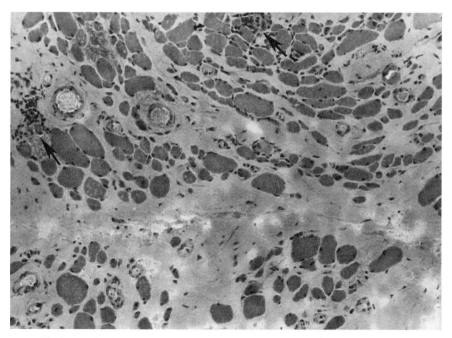

Figure 4-13. Muscle biopsy specimen from the supraspinatus muscle of a 17-year-old man with facioscapulohumeral dystrophy. This specimen shows marked variation in myofiber size, focal infiltrates of inflammatory cells *(arrows),* and severe fibrosis. A previous biopsy specimen from his deltoid showed no significant abnormalities. H&E, ×215.

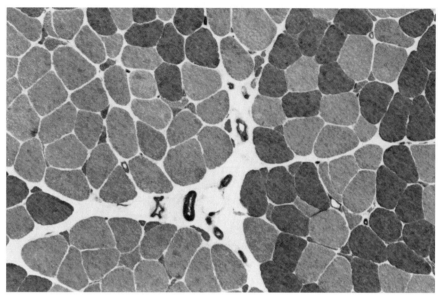

Figure 4-14. Fiber-type grouping and small angular denervated myofibers in a 10-year-old girl with a neurogenic facioscapulohumeral syndrome. ATPase, pH 10.4, × 200.

LIMB GIRDLE DYSTROPHY

The term "limb girdle dystrophy" is used to designate a diverse group of diseases that are characterized by slowly progressive proximal muscular weakness.[1,34] The disorders begin in the second and third decades and eventually lead to severe disability in about 20 years. They tend to spare the facial muscles. All of the disorders included under this heading are rare and most appear to be inherited as autosomal-recessive traits. Among the more distinct entities included in this rather heterogeneous group of disorders are a pelvifemoral dystrophy and a scapulohumeral dystrophy. Many cases formerly classified as limb girdle dystrophy have been reclassified as Becker dystrophy, spinal muscular atrophies, metabolic myopathies, and congenital myopathies.

The scapulohumeral form is manifested by slowly progressive weakness of the upper arm, especially the biceps, and the muscles of the shoulder girdle. The proximal lower limb and pelvic girdle muscles may be affected later in the course of the disease. As with facioscapulohumeral dystrophy, the deltoids and forearm muscles are relatively spared. The disease is steadily progressive but the serum CK levels are usually only mildly elevated.

The pelvifemoral form of limb girdle dystrophy is rare and poorly characterized. The patients included in this category pursue a slowly progressive course. Many of the cases formerly included in this group have been reclassified in more recent years.

In view of the diversity of disorders included under the heading of limb girdle dystrophy, it is not surprising that the morphologic findings are relatively nonspecific. Muscle specimens from these patients show changes of a chronic myopathy and the severity of these alterations vary with the stage of the disease.[35] The milder and presumably earlier changes include variation in myofiber size (Fig. 4–15), and increased numbers of internal nuclei. Some cases show type I myofiber predominance. With progression of the diseases, fiber splitting becomes prominent. There may be groups of both large and small myofibers of a single fiber type encased by the proliferated endomysial connective tissue. The larger myofibers often show distortions of the intermyofibrillar network. These alterations are best seen with the NADH–TR reaction. Numerous ring fibers and occasional lobulated fibers also may be present.[31] Hyalinized and necrotic fibers are infrequent and inflammation is sparse.

OCULOPHARYNGEAL DYSTROPHY

Oculopharyngeal dystrophy is an autosomal-dominant disorder that is characterized by ptosis and dysphagia.[36] These manifestations become apparent relatively late in life, generally after the fourth decade, and may be accompanied by mild weakness of proximal limb muscles. Most of the familial cases of this uncommon disorder have been described in French or French–Canadian individuals. Familial cases also have been reported among Spanish–Americans in the western part of the United States.[14]

Muscle specimens from these patients have shown increased variation in myofiber size with scattered small angular myofibers. Many of the atrophic

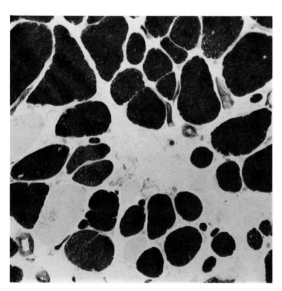

Figure 4–15. Muscle biopsy specimen from a 40-year-old man with proximal muscle weakness progressing slowly over the past 20 years. Neither parents nor four siblings were similarly affected. Clinically the patient was thought to have limb girdle dystrophy. The morphologic changes are not diagnostic. ATPase, pH 9.4 ×200.

fibers are type I myofibers. The type II myofibers may show hypertrophy. Moth-eaten and whorled myofibers also may be seen. A commonly encountered histologic feature is the presence of "rimmed vacuoles," similar to those seen in inclusion body myositis. These small vacuoles are found predominantly in atrophic type I myofibers. The vacuoles contain finely granular material that stains blue with H&E and red with the modified trichrome procedure. Occasionally, the granular contents appear to be "smeared" onto the adjacent intact portions of the affected myofiber. Although rimmed vacuoles are often seen in oculopharyngeal dystrophy, similar vacuoles have been encountered in a wide variety of other neuromuscular diseases.[37] The rimmed vacuoles must be distinguished from "ragged-red" fibers. When abundant "ragged-red" fibers are encountered in a patient with an ocular myopathy, the Kearns–Shy syndrome must be considered in the differential diagnosis.

Several authors[38–40] have described nuclear inclusions composed of thin filaments or tubules measuring 7 to 9 μm in diameter, as another feature of oculopharyngeal dystrophy. The specificity of this feature has been challenged.[41] We have encountered similar intranuclear filamentous inclusions in polymyositis (see Fig. 3–6) and facioscapulohumeral dystrophy.

CONGENITAL MUSCULAR DYSTROPHY

The congenital muscular dystrophies are a heterogeneous group of ill-defined neuromuscular disorders. Clinically, the patients are characterized by generalized weakness and hypotonia from birth. Some also have facial weakness similar to patients with facioscapulohumeral dystrophy. The course of the disease is variable. Some patients pursue a slowly progressive course while others have a static course or even show mild improvement in childhood. Many have contractures at birth or develop them soon thereafter. Electromyographic studies show "myopathic" features and the CK levels are normal to moderately elevated. Most of the cases appear to be inherited as an autosomal-recessive trait although other modes of inheritance have been suggested. Because of the variability in the course of the disease, some authors, such as Zellweger et al., have divided the cases into a severe form[42] and a more benign form.[43] These clinically disparate entities were grouped together largely on the basis of morphologic findings in muscle biopsy specimens. The alterations consisted predominantly of increased variation in myofiber size, numerous internalized nuclei, and prominent endomysial fibrosis. The earlier morphologic studies were performed almost entirely on paraffin-embedded sections. It has been suggested[44] that at least some of these patients might have been classified differently by histochemical studies on frozen sections.

A more recent study of congenital muscular dystrophy by Lazaro et al.[45] described the morphologic features as consisting of increased variation in myofiber size with only rare degenerating myofibers, occasional internalized nuclei, type I myofiber predominance, and very extensive endomysial fibrosis with adipose infiltration. In contrast to most other muscle disorders, some of these patients showed marked degeneration of intrafusal myofibers and fibrosis of the spindle capsule.

Another, probably distinct disorder, that is often included among the congenital muscular dystrophies is Fukuyama muscular dystrophy. This autosomal-recessive disorder was originally described in Japan but has now been observed in other parts of the world.[46-48] In addition to muscular weakness, the affected individuals have involvement of the central nervous system. This is manifested by mental retardation and seizures. Neuropathologic studies have demonstrated a wide variety of central nervous system lesions. These have included lobar polymicrogyria, pachygyria, and cerebellar polymicrogyria.[49] Other patients have shown agenesis of the corpus callosum and partial fusion of the frontal lobes. Some authors have suggested that this complex of central nervous system and musculoskeletal abnormalities may be the result of intrauterine infection rather than a muscular dystrophy.

References

1. Walton JN, Gardner-Medwin D: Progressive muscular dystrophy and the myotonic disorders. In Walton JN (ed): Disorders of Voluntary Muscle, 4th ed. Edinburgh, Churchill Livingstone, 1981, pp 481–524.
2. Gomez MR, Engel AG, Dewald G, Peterson HA: Failure of inactivation of Duchenne dystrophy X-chromosome in one of female identical twins. Neurology 27:537–541, 1977.
3. Olson BJ, Fenichel GM: Progressive muscle disease in a young woman with family history of Duchenne's muscular dystrophy. Arch Neurol 39:378–380, 1982.
4. Dubowitz V: The muscular dystrophies. In Dubowitz V (ed): Muscle Disorders in Childhood. London, Saunders, 1978, pp 19–69.
5. Lane RJM, Gardner-Medwin D, Roses AD: Electrocardiographic abnormalities in carriers of Duchenne muscular dystrophy. Neurology 30:497–501, 1980.
6. Crisp DE, Ziter FA, Bray PF: Diagnostic delay in Duchenne's muscular dystrophy. JAMA 247:478–480, 1982.
7. Mahoney MJ, Haseltine FP, Hobbins JC, et al.: Prenatal diagnosis of Duchenne's muscular dystrophy. N Engl J Med 297:968–973, 1977.
8. Globus MS, Stephens JD, Mahoney MJ, et al.: Failure of fetal creatine phosphokinase as a diagnostic indicator of Duchenne muscular dystrophy. N Engl J Med 300:860–861, 1979.
9. Bodensteiner JB, Engel AG: Intracellular calcium accumulation in Duchenne dystrophy and other myopathies: A study of 567,000 muscle fibers in 114 biopsies. Neurology 28:439–446, 1978.
10. Mokri B, Engel AG: Duchenne dystrophy: Electron microscopic findings pointing to a basic or early abnormality in the plasma membrane of the muscle fiber. Neurology 25:1111–1120, 1975.
11. Wakayama Y, Bonilla E, Schotland DL: Muscle plasma membrane abnormalities in infants with Duchenne muscular dystrophy. Neurology 33:1368–1370, 1983.
12. Carpenter S, Karpati G: Duchenne muscular dystrophy: Plasma membrane loss initiates muscle cell necrosis unless it is repaired. Brain 102:147–161, 1979.

13. Schmalbruch H: Segmental fiber breakdown and defects of the plasmalemma in diseased human muscles. Acta Neuropathol 33:129–141, 1975.

14. Dubowitz V, Brooke MH: Muscle Biopsy: A Modern Approach. London, Saunders, 1973, pp 169–178.

15. Miike T: Maturational defect of regenerating muscle fibers in cases with Duchenne and congenital muscular dystrophies. Muscle Nerve 6:545–552, 1983.

16. Hathaway PW, Engel WK, Zellweger H: Experimental myopathy after microarterial embolization: Comparison with childhood X-linked pseudohypertrophic muscular dystrophy. Arch Neurol 22:365–378, 1970.

17. Jerusalem F, Engel AG, Gomez MR: Duchenne dystrophy. I. Morphometric study of the muscle microvasculature. Brain 97:115–122, 1974.

18. Sakakibara H, Engel AG, Lambert EH: Duchenne dystrophy: Ultrastructural localization of the acetylcholine receptor and intracellular microelectrode studies of neuromuscular transmission. Neurology 27:741–745, 1977.

19. Rowland LP: Biochemistry of muscle membranes in Duchenne muscular dystrophy. Muscle Nerve 3:3–20, 1980.

20. Griggs RC, Rennie MJ: Muscle wasting in muscular dystrophy: Decreased protein synthesis or increased degradation? Ann Neurol 13:125–132, 1982.

21. Bradley WG, Keleman J: Genetic counseling in Duchenne muscular dystrophy (editorial). Muscle Nerve 2:325–328, 1979.

22. Percy ME, Andrews DF, Thompson MW: Serum creatine kinase in the detection of Duchenne muscular dystrophy carriers: Effects of season and multiple testing. Muscle Nerve 5:58–64, 1982.

23. Becker PE, Kiener F: Eine neue X-chromosomale Muskeldystrophie. Arch Psychiatr Nervenkr 193:427–448, 1955.

24. Becker PE: Two new families of benign sex-linked recessive muscular dystrophy. Rev Can Biol 21:551–566, 1962.

25. Bradley WG, Jones MZ, Mussini JM, Fawcett PRW: Becker-type muscular dystrophy. Muscle Nerve 1:111–132, 1978.

26. Ringel SP, Carroll JE, Schold SC: The spectrum of mild X-linked recessive muscular dystrophy. Arch Neurol 34:408–416, 1977.

27. Hastings BA, Groothuis DR, Vick NA: Dominantly inherited pseudohypertrophic muscular dystrophy with internalized capillaries. Arch Neurol 37:709–714, 1980.

28. Goebel HH, Prange H, Gullotta F, et al.: Becker's X-linked muscular dystrophy: Histological, enzyme-histochemical, and ultrastructural studies of two cases, originally reported by Becker. Acta Neuropathol 46:69–77, 1979.

29. ten Houten R, De Visser M: Histopathological findings in Becker-type muscular dystrophy. Arch Neurol 41:729–733, 1984.

30. Brooke MH: A Clinician's View of Neuromuscular Diseases. Baltimore, Williams & Wilkins, 1977, pp 109–116.

31. Bethlem J, Van Wijngaarden GK, De Jong J: The incidence of lobulated fibres in the facioscapulohumeral type of muscular dystrophy and the limb-girdle syndrome. J Neurol Sci 18:351–358, 1973.

32. Munsat TL, Piper D, Cancilla P, Mednick J: Inflammatory myopathy with facioscapulohumeral distribution. Neurology 22:335–347, 1972.

33. Kazakov VM, Bogorodinsky DK, Znoyko ZV, Skorometz AA: The facio-scapulo-limb (or the facioscapulohumeral) type of muscular dystrophy. Eur Neurol 11:236–260, 1974.

34. Bradley WG: The limb-girdle syndromes. In Vinken PJ, Bruyn GW (eds): Handbook of Clinical Neurology. Amsterdam, North-Holland, 1979, Vol 40, pp 433–469.

35. Schmalbruch H: The muscular dystrophies. In Walton JN (ed): Disorders of Voluntary Muscle, 4th ed. Edinburgh, Churchill Livingstone, 1981, pp 235–265.

36. Victor M, Hayes R, Adams RD: Oculopharyngeal muscular dystrophy. A familial disease of late life characterized by dysphagia and progressive ptosis of the eyelids. N Engl J Med 267:1267–1272, 1962.

37. Fukuhara N, Kumamoto T, Tsubaki T: Rimmed vacuoles. Acta Neuropathol 51:229–235, 1980.

38. Tome FMS, Fardeau M: Nuclear inclusions in oculopharyngeal dystrophy. Acta Neuropathol 49:85–87, 1980.

39. Martin JJR, Ceuterick CM, Mercelis RJ: Nuclear inclusions in oculopharyngeal muscular dystrophy. Muscle Nerve 5:735–737, 1982.

40. Coquet M, Vallat JM, Vital C, et al.: Nuclear inclusions in oculopharyngeal dystrophy. J Neurol Sci 60:151–156, 1983.

41. Smith TW, Chad D: Intranuclear inclusions in oculopharyngeal dystrophy. Muscle Nerve 7:339–340, 1984.

42. Zellweger H, Afifi A, McCormick WF, Mergner W: Severe congenital muscular dystrophy. Am J Dis Child 114:591–602, 1967.

43. Zellweger H, Afifi A, McCormick WF, Mergner W: Benign congenital muscular dystrophy: A special form of congenital hypotonia. Clin Pediatr 6:655–663, 1967.

44. Brooke MH, Carroll JE, Ringel SP: Congenital hypotonia revisited. Muscle Nerve 2:84–100, 1979.

45. Lazaro RP, Fenichel GM, Kilroy AW: Congenital muscular dystrophy: Case reports and reappraisal. Muscle Nerve 2:349–355, 1979.

46. Nonaka I, Chou SM: Congenital muscular dystrophy. In Vinken PJ, Bruyn GW (eds): Handbook of Clinical Neurology. Amsterdam, North-Holland, 1979, Vol 41, pp 27–50.

47. Nonaka I, Sugita H, Takada K, Kumagai K: Muscle histochemistry in congenital muscular dystrophy with central nervous system involvement. Muscle Nerve 5:102–106, 1982.

48. Dambska M, Wisniewski K, Sher J, Solish G: Cerebro-oculo-muscular syndrome: A variant of Fukuyama congenital cerebromuscular dystrophy. Clin Neuropathol 1:93–98, 1982.

49. Takada K, Nakamura H, Tanaka J: Cortical dysplasia in congenital muscular dystrophy with central nervous system involvement (Fukuyama type). J Neuropathol Exp Neurol 43:395–407, 1984.

chapter 5

Myotonic Dystrophy and the Genetic Myotonias

The conditions considered in this chapter have myotonia as one of their major clinical manifestations. *Myotonia* is the persistence of muscle contractions after voluntary efforts or direct stimulation have ceased. Clinically myotonia can be manifested in several ways. For example, it may be apparent in the form of abnormally slow relaxation of a tight grip, or the delayed opening of tightly closed eyelids. Myotonia also can be demonstrated as an abnormally persistent dimpling following the direct percussion of a muscle. In addition to the visible manifestations, electromyographic studies disclose characteristic repetitive discharges that gradually decrease in amplitude. When demonstrated acoustically, these high-frequency discharges are often described as sounding similar to a "dive bomber." Myotonia may be detected electrically even when it is otherwise not apparent. The abnormal electrical discharges tend to be more severe in distal muscles.

Myotonia is thought to be a manifestation of muscle membrane abnormalities. It persists after nerve section and pharmacologic blockade of neuromuscular transmission. No consistent morphologic abnormalities have been demonstrated at the neuromuscular junctions although some studies have shown elongation of the synaptic region with an increase in the number of terminal axonal expansions.[1] Biochemical studies have suggested abnormalities of chloride conductance[2] or abnormal fluidity of the muscle membranes.[3] Myotonia has been produced experimentally in laboratory animals intoxicated with various drugs.

There are at least three genetically determined neuromuscular diseases that have myotonia as one of their major clinical manifestations. These are myotonic dystrophy, myotonia congenita, and paramyotonia. Myotonic dystrophy, paramyotonia, and some cases of myotonia congenita are inherited as autosomal-dominant traits with variable penetrance. Other than sharing myotonia and having a similar genetic basis, these diseases are quite different. In addition to these diseases, electrical myotonia is occasionally demonstrable in patients with various glycogenoses such as adult acid maltase deficiency.[4]

MYOTONIC DYSTROPHY

Myotonic dystrophy is a relatively common disorder with an estimated prevalence of 3 to 5/100,000 individuals. The disease usually does not become symptomatic until adult life; however, with careful examination the disease often can be detected in childhood. Even infantile and congenital cases of myotonic dystrophy are well documented. The disease is highly variable in its expression and many cases remain subclinical. When symptomatic, the patients often complain of weakness, especially of the distal arm and hand muscles, difficulty in walking, and a tendency to fall. Even the latter complaints are the result of distal leg and foot weakness. The weakness is slowly progressive and eventually can lead to severe disability. The patients also have weakness of face and neck muscles. This may be manifested by ptosis, facial diplegia, gaping mouth, and forward tilting of the head. Oropharyngeal muscle weakness may result in dysarthria and dysphagia. Atrophy of the face, temporal, and neck muscles along with frontal baldness in men, imparts a stereotyped appearance to many of these patients. The myotonia generally causes fewer symptoms than the weakness. Stiffness and difficulty relaxing contracted muscles are less common complaints. The myotonia is aggravated by cold and relieved by exercise.

Myotonic dystrophy affects many other organ systems in addition to the skeletal muscles.[5] Cardiac involvement is generally manifested only by electrocardiographic abnormalities. In some patients, however, heart failure and sudden death have been attributed to the associated conduction defects. The cardiac involvement poses a special problem during surgery. Patients with myotonic dystrophy may be abnormally sensitive to induction agents and anesthetics. Adverse reactions may occur even when the individuals previously have tolerated the same agents. The major morphologic abnormality that has been seen in the hearts of patients with myotonic dystrophy is interstitial fibrosis.

Cataracts are a common finding in patients with myotonic dystrophy, however, slit lamp examination may be necessary to demonstrate their presence. The cataracts most often involve the posterior and subcapsular regions of the lens. In some individuals, they may be the only evidence of the disease. Rarely, they are present even in infancy.

Contraction of smooth muscle in the gastrointestinal and genitourinary tracts is impaired and leads to bowel and bladder dysfunction. The most striking genitourinary abnormality is, however, testicular atrophy. Histologic study of the atrophic gonads shows hyalinization of the seminiferous tubules. Women with myotonic dystrophy may have menstrual irregularities and reduced fertility but the ovaries are histologically unremarkable.

Several minor skeletal abnormalities are encountered frequently. Many patients, especially children with this disease, have small mandibles and micrognathia. Hyperostosis frontalis, unusually large paranasal sinuses, and a relatively small sella turcica are among the other common skeletal anomalies.

There is an increased prevalence of mental retardation and deviant behavior among patients with myotonic dystrophy. Morphologic studies of the nervous system have failed, however, to reveal significant correlative abnormalities. Mild anomalies of gyral configuration have been reported in some patients. Culebras et al.[6] and Wisniewski et al.[7] have described small eosinophilic intracytoplasmic inclusions within occasional thalamic neurons. Ultrastructurally the inclusions appear to be composed of parallel fibrils that vary in their degree of osmiophilia. The relation between these inclusions and myotonic dystrophy remains unclear. Similar inclusions also have been found in occasional individuals without this disease.

Serum immunoglobulin levels in patients with myotonic dystrophy are generally lower than normal. The immunoglobulin abnormality has been attributed to increased catabolism of the serum protein, however, the site of the enhanced degradation remains unknown. Silver et al.[8] investigated the distribution of the immunoglobulins in skeletal muscle but were unable to relate the decreased serum levels to binding at sites of myofiber necrosis. Patients with myotonic dystrophy frequently have an abnormal glucose tolerance test and an excessive insulin response to glucose challenge. This has been attributed to decreased insulin receptor affinity.[9]

Because of the multiple systems involved in myotonic dystrophy, attempts have been made to investigate the fundamental cellular abnormalities by studying the structure and growth characteristics of fibroblasts in tissue cultures. Despite earlier reports to the contrary, recent studies have failed to demonstrate any consistent morphologic abnormalities or differences in the incorporation of radioactive sulfate.[10]

NEONATAL MYOTONIC DYSTROPHY

In the neonate, congenital myotonic dystrophy may be manifested by severe hypotonia, facial diplegia, and respiratory difficulties. Some of the infants have such severe oropharyngeal weakness that they are unable to suck or swallow. These infants also have a wide spectrum of visceral and somatic anomalies involving the skin, eyes, heart, genitourinary system, and endocrine system. They may have talipes equinovarus, anomalies of the ribs, and abnormalities of the diaphragm. Some of the anomalies, such as nesidioblastosis, persistent renal blastemas, cryptorchidism, and patent ductus arteriosus have been interpreted as evidence of maturational arrest.[11]

Congenital myotonic dystrophy occurs only in infants who have inherited the mutant gene from their mother. Some workers have interpreted this observation as evidence that congenital myotonic dystrophy results from the interaction of the mutant gene and the abnormal intrauterine environment in the affected mother. Accurate diagnosis of the disease in infancy may depend on evaluation and diagnosis of the maternal disease. Electromyographic studies on these infants may fail to disclose the characteristic electrical manifestations of myotonia.

HISTOPATHOLOGY

Muscle specimens from patients with myotonic dystrophy show a wide spectrum of morphologic changes. Although these changes do not correlate closely with the stage or the severity of the clinical disease, there is predictable variation according to the age of the patient.

Usually specimens from adults and older children show increased variation in myofiber size. This is due to the presence of moderately to severely atrophic myofibers that are predominantly type I myofibers and relatively few, if any, hypertrophied myofibers (Figs. 5-1 through 5-4). Selective atrophy of type I myofibers, although variable in degree, is one of the most characteristic morphologic alterations of this disease. Some of the atrophic myofibers may be reduced to mere knots of sarcolemmal nuclei. Although these fibers resemble denervation myofibers, studies with alpha-bungarotoxin have failed to show spread of acetylcholine receptor. Therefore, they are thought to arise through processes other than denervation.[12]

Internal nuclei are often markedly increased in number (Fig. 5-5). When

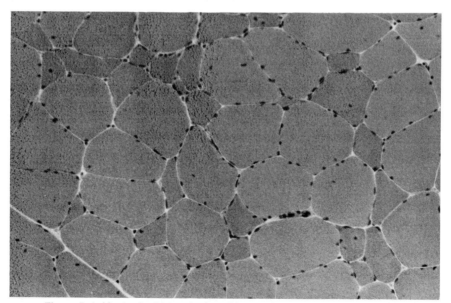

Figure 5-1. Myotonic dystrophy in a 34-year-old man. Moderately atrophic myofibers are scattered individually and aggregated in small groups. H&E, ×170.

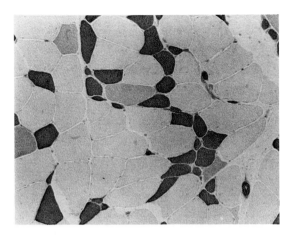

Figure 5-2. The atrophic myofibers are predominantly type
I myofibers *(dark)*. ATPase,
preincubated at pH 4.3, × 120.

the muscle is viewed in transverse sections, these nuclei appear scattered about
the interior of the myofibers but often appear to be aligned in chains when
longitudinal sections are examined. The internal nuclei may be found in both
normal-sized and atrophic myofibers of both types. Occasionally, the internal
nuclei are found predominantly in the mildly to moderately atrophic type I
myofibers (Fig. 5-6). Electron microscopy often discloses small collections of
vesicles and electron-dense bodies (Fig. 5-7) near the internal and subsarcolemmal nuclei. These are thought to be lysosomes.[1,13,14] They may be sufficiently numerous to result in increased acid phosphatase activity that can be
demonstrated histochemically.

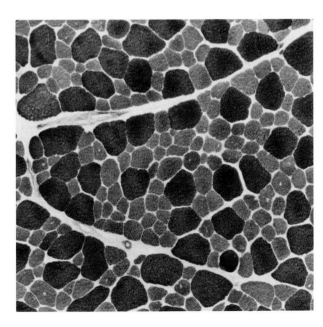

Figure 5-3. Myotonic
dystrophy in a 12-year-
old boy, brother of the
patient shown in Figure
5-4. Note the moderate
atrophy affecting vir-
tually all of the type I
myofibers *(light fibers)*.
ATPase, pH 9.4, × 170.

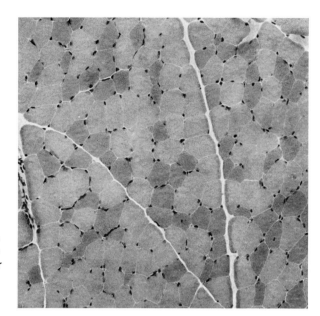

Figure 5-4. Myotonic dystrophy in an 8-year-old boy, brother of patient shown in Figure 5-3. Note the mild atrophy of type I myofibers *(darker fibers)* evident even at this early age. Trichrome, × 200.

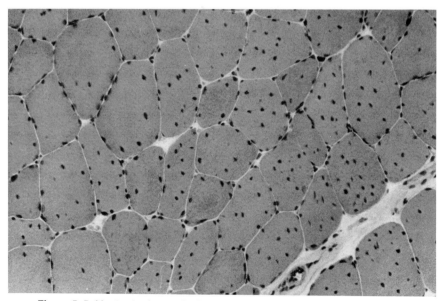

Figure 5-5. Myotonic dystrophy in a 25-year-old man. Note the marked increase in the number of internal nuclei. H&E, × 170.

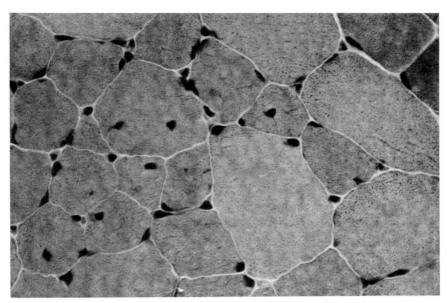

Figure 5-6. Occasionally internal nuclei are encountered, predominantly in the mildly to moderately atrophic type I myofibers (same patient as in Fig. 5-3). Trichrome, ×510.

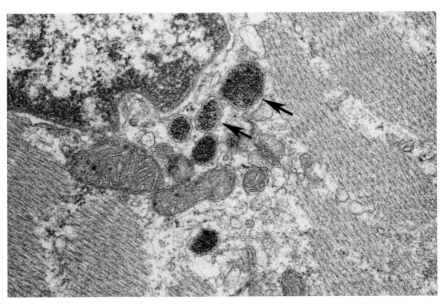

Figure 5-7. Myotonic dystrophy in a 48-year-old woman. This electron micrograph shows electron-dense vesicles *(arrows)* near the nucleus. These are thought to be lysosomes and may be sufficiently numerous to produce enhanced acid phosphatase activity that can be demonstrated histochemically. ×60,000.

Other histopathologic features of myotonic dystrophy are the presence of sarcoplasmic masses and ring fibers. The sarcoplasmic masses are peripheral bands or foci of abnormal homogeneous-appearing sarcoplasm. These areas may partially or completely encircle the affected myofibers (Fig. 5–8). The abnormal sarcoplasm stains bluish with H&E, red with trichrome, and dark blue with the NADH–TR reaction. By electron microscopy, the sarcoplasmic masses correspond to areas in which there are numerous glycogen granules, mitochondria, ribosomes, and dense bodies. Some of the mitochondria may show structural abnormalities including intracristal paracrystalline arrays. The sarcoplasmic masses are generally devoid of organized contractile elements. Occasionally small bundles of filaments and clumps of osmiophilic granular material resembling disorganized Z-discs may be seen. Rarely, the sarcoplasmic masses contain cytoplasmic bodies.[1] Sarcoplasmic masses may be found in other diseases but are especially numerous in myotonic dystrophy.

Ring fibers, otherwise designated as *ringbinden* or *spiral annulets,* are often abundant in specimens from patients with myotonic dystrophy. They appear as bundles of myofibrils that encircle or spiral around the myofiber as a helix perpendicular to its long axis (Fig. 5–9). Rarely, the aberrant myofibrils appear

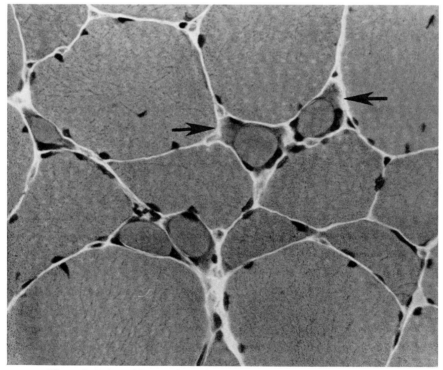

Figure 5-8. Atrophic type I myofibers containing sarcoplasmic masses *(arrows)* from a patient with myotonic dystrophy. H&E, ×510.

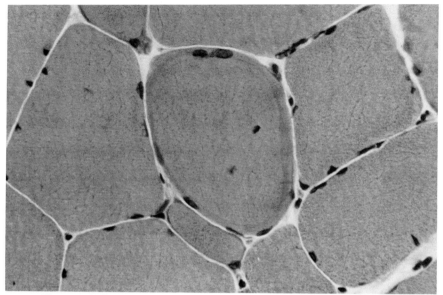

Figure 5-9. Ring fibers in a patient with myotonic dystrophy. Note the bundle of aberrant myofibrils that encircles the fiber in the center of the figure. H&E, ×510.

to cross the interior of the myofiber. Some ring fibers occur in association with sarcoplasmic masses. Under these circumstances, the aberrant myofibrils may be located immediately beneath the abnormal sarcoplasm. Ring fibers can be seen with a variety of stains but are often most clearly seen with the PAS technique. In many instances, they can be detected more readily by examining sections with polarized light. This causes the bundles of aberrant myofibrils to appear bright against a dark background. In paraffin-embedded sections, ring fibers are best demonstrated with the trichrome and PTAH stains. As with sarcoplasmic masses, ring fibers are abundant in specimens from patients with myotonic dystrophy but are not restricted to this condition. In some instances, ring fibers appear to result from artifactual contraction of the muscle biopsy specimen.

Necrotic myofibers and fibers undergoing myophagocytosis are not common findings in specimens from patients with myotonic dystrophy. Inflammation is generally minimal, and when present is largely confined to areas adjacent to necrotic myofibers. Endomysial fibrosis is variable. It is most pronounced among the severely atrophic myofibers in older patients.

There are numerous additional nonspecific degenerative changes that are best seen by electron microscopy. Honeycomb arrays, derived from the T-tubules, and dilatation and proliferation of the sarcoplasmic reticulum may be prominent. Some fibers may show conspicuous duplication of the triads. Nemaline rods may be seen in some of the more severely atrophic myofibers (Fig.

5–10). Tome and Fardeau[15] have described "fingerprint bodies" in three patients with myotonic dystrophy. These bodies were virtually identical to the structures described by Engel et al.[16] in so-called "fingerprint myopathy."

Specimens from infants with congenital myotonic dystrophy are highly variable in appearance. Some appear nearly normal while others show preferential atrophy of type I or II myofibers, along with increased numbers of internal nuclei (Figs. 5–11 and 5–12). Since myofibers from these infants are quite small, the internal location of the nuclei may be appreciated more readily in epoxy-embedded sections and by electron microscopy (Fig. 5–13) than in frozen sections. These fibers may resemble the fibers seen in centronuclear myopathy.[17] Argov et al.[18] have reported a patient with congenital myotonic dystrophy with type IIB myofiber deficiency and predominance of small type I myofibers. Histologically, this case closely resembled congenital fiber-type disproportion. Lipofuscin, seen as autofluorescent deposits, may be increased sufficiently in infantile cases, to mimic those seen in patients with ceroid-lipofuscinosis.[14]

Muscle spindles frequently show morphologic abnormalities in patients with myotonic dystrophy.[19] Swash[20] found abnormalities in about 40 percent of spindles and noted that they were more prominent in spindles from distal muscles. The abnormalities included excessive numbers of intrafusal fibers, among which there were degenerative changes. These fibers showed fiber splitting, necrosis, and regeneration. Some of the spindle capsules showed fibrosis. The pathogenesis of these alterations is unknown. Recent studies in patients

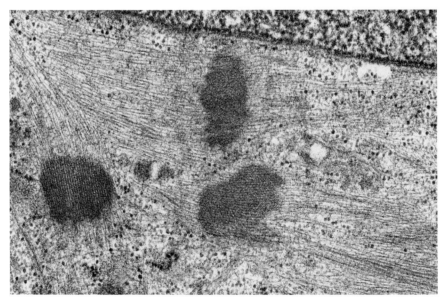

Figure 5–10. Small nemaline rods are seen by electron microscopy in an atrophic myofiber. ×60,000.

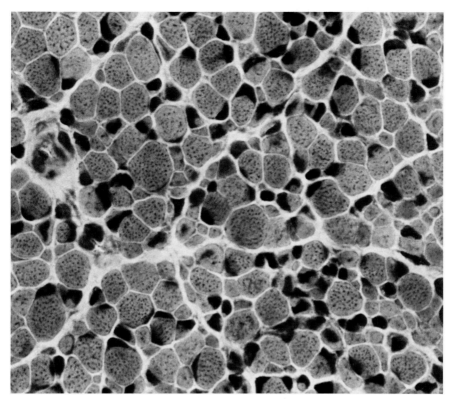

Figure 5-11. Muscle biopsy specimen from a neonate with congenital myotonic dystrophy. The mother and paternal siblings had typical myotonic dystrophy. This infant was hypotonic and had severe respiratory difficulties prior to his death at 3 days of age. Note the numerous very small myofibers. Trichrome, ×820.

with myotonia congenita failed to disclose comparable spindle abnormalities.[21] This suggests that the degenerative changes in the intrafusal fibers in myotonic dystrophy are an integral part of the disease and not merely the result of the myotonia.

MYOTONIA CONGENITA

This disorder is much rarer than myotonic dystrophy, however, several very large kindreds have been reported. The classic description of this disease was published in 1876 by Thomsen[22] who himself had the disease. His report was based on personal observations and 20 members of his family spanning a period of four generations. The disease is regarded as genetically heterogeneous. Becker[23] delineated an autosomal-recessive form that in some areas, e.g., Ger-

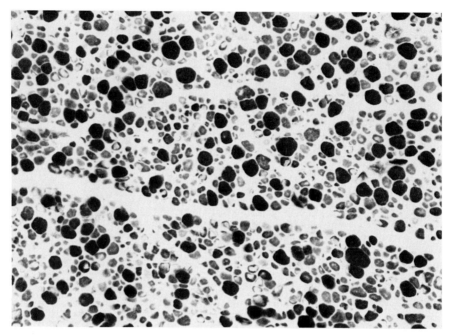

Figure 5-12. Congenital myotonic dystrophy. Unlike adults and older children with myotonic dystrophy, most of the severely atrophic fibers in this specimen are type II myofibers *(light)*. ATPase, preincubated at pH 4.3, ×510.

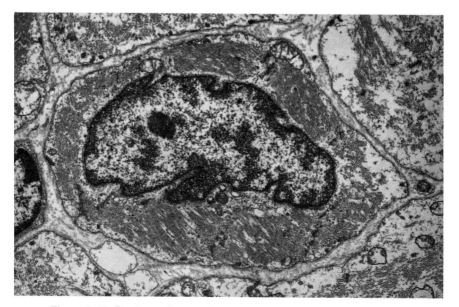

Figure 5-13. Electron micrographs showing the central location of the nucleus in one of the atrophic myofibers. ×14,000.

many, is more common than the classic autosomal-dominant form. Both of these genotypes have been further subdivided into additional variants. The dominant forms usually become evident in infancy or early childhood while the recessive forms often have a later onset of symptoms. These may be more severe than in the dominant forms and affect the legs more than the upper extremities.[24-26] All forms of the disease cause stiffness that is accentuated by rest and relieved by exercise. Some of the autosomal-dominant forms are further characterized by cramps and sensitivity to cold. Both genotypes lead to generalized muscular hypertrophy. Eventually, mild wasting of the distal portions of the extremities may develop. In all forms, the myotonia is readily demonstrated by physical examination and electrophysiologic studies. Serum CK levels may be mildly elevated. In contrast to myotonic dystrophy, other organ systems are spared.

Histologic examination of muscle specimens from patients with myotonia congenita reveals changes that are much less prominent than those usually seen in specimens from patients wth myotonic dystrophy. The myofibers show mildly increased variation in size due to the presence of both atrophic and hypertrophied fibers. The hypertrophied fibers are larger and more numerous in the autosomal-recessive variants. Increased numbers of internal nuclei and rare necrotic myofibers are seen in both genotypes. Tubular aggregates are more frequently encountered in specimens from patients with the autosomal-dominant forms.[24] In some but not all cases of myotonia congenita, there is a striking deficiency of type IIB myofibers.[27] Electron microscopy shows only mild, nonspecific alterations. In contrast to myotonic dystrophy, ring fibers and sarcoplasmic masses are rare and muscle spindles are morphologically unremarkable.[21]

PARAMYOTONIA CONGENITA

This is a rare and somewhat controversial myotonic disorder. It was originally described in 1886 by Eulenburg[28] who reported 26 cases in six generations of a single family. The disease is inherited as an autosomal-dominant trait with a high degree of penetrance. Manifestations of the disease are evident from infancy. It is characterized by the development of stiffness followed by weakness upon exposure to cold. Both the stiffness and weakness subside with warming.[5] The myotonia may be exacerbated by exercise. Some authors have suggested that this disease should be regarded as a variant of hyperkalemic periodic paralysis. Pharmacologic studies, however, have shown striking differences between these disorders. In contrast to hyperkalemic periodic paralysis, the administration of potassium has been shown to exacerbate the myotonia but not to precipitate weakness. Conversely, the administration of acetazolamide has been shown to ameliorate the myotonia but to cause profound weakness in at least some patients with paramyotonia.[29]

Histologic examination of muscle specimens from patients with paramyotonia have disclosed diverse findings. Some specimens have shown only minimal alterations consisting of mildly increased variation in myofiber size and a mild increase in the number of internal nuclei. Other patients have shown more marked variation in myofiber size due to the presence of both hypertrophied and atrophic myofibers. Internal nuclei may be quite numerous and may be accompanied by vacuoles, tubular aggregates, and subsarcolemmal masses. Because of the overlap with hyperkalemic periodic paralysis, it is difficult to evaluate the relatively limited reports of the morphologic findings in this disorder.

References

1. Schroder JM, Adams RD: The ultrastructural morphology of the muscle fiber in myotonic dystrophy. Acta Neuropathol 10:218–241, 1968.
2. Barchi RL: Myotonia: An evaluation of the chloride hypothesis. Arch Neurol 32:175–180, 1975.
3. Roses AD, Harper PS, Bossen EH: Myotonic muscular dystrophy. In Vinken PJ, Bruyn GW (eds): Handbook of Clinical Neurology. Amsterdam, North-Holland, 1979, Vol 40, pp 485–532.
4. McComas CF, Schochet SS Jr, Morris HH III, et al.: The constellation of adult acid maltase deficiency. Clin Neuropathol 2:182–187, 1983.
5. Zellweger H, Ionasescu V: Myotonic dystrophy and its differential diagnosis. Acta Neurol Scand 49 (Suppl 55):5–28, 1973.
6. Culebras A, Feldman RG, Merk F: Cytoplasmic inclusion bodies within neurons of the thalamus in myotonic dystrophy. J Neurol Sci 19:319–329, 1973.
7. Wisniewski HM, Berry K, Spiro AJ: Ultrastructure of thalamic neuronal inclusions in myotonic dystrophy. J Neurol Sci 24:321–329, 1975.
8. Silver MM, Banerjee D, Hudson AJ: Segmental myofiber necrosis in myotonic dystrophy: An immunoperoxidase study of immunoglobulins in skeletal muscle. Am J Pathol 112:294–301, 1983.
9. Stuart CA, Armstrong RM, Provow SA, Plishker GA: Insulin resistance in patients with myotonic dystrophy. Neurology 33:679–685, 1983.
10. Hartwig GB, Miller SE, Frost AP, Roses AD: Myotonic muscular dystrophy: Morphology, histochemistry, and growth characteristics of cultured skin fibroblasts. Muscle Nerve 5:125–130, 1982.
11. Young SK, Gang DL, Zalneraitis EL, Krishnamoorthy KS: Dysmaturation in infants of mothers with myotonic dystrophy. Arch Neurol 38:716–719, 1981.
12. Drachman DB, Fambrough DM: Are muscle fibers denervated in myotonic dystrophy? Arch Neurol 33:485–488, 1976.
13. Klinkerfuss GH: An electron microscopic study of myotonic dystrophy. Arch Neurol 16:181–193, 1967.
14. Karpati G, Carpenter S, Watters GV, et al.: Infantile myotonic dystrophy: Histochemical and electron microscopic features in skeletal muscle. Neurology 23:1066–1077, 1973.
15. Tome FMS, Fardeau M: "Fingerprint inclusions" in muscle fibres in dystrophia myotonica. Acta Neuropathol 24:62–67, 1973.
16. Engel AG, Angelini C, Gomez MR: Fingerprint body myopathy. A newly recognized congenital muscle disease. Proc Mayo Clin 47:377–388, 1972.

17. Sarnat HG, Silbert SW: Maturational arrest of fetal muscle in neonatal myotonic dystrophy. Arch Neurol 33:466–474, 1976.
18 Argov Z, Gardner-Medwin D, Johnson MA, Mastaglia FL: Congenital myotonic dystrophy: Fiber type abnormalities in two cases. Arch Neurol 37:693–696, 1980.
19. Heene R: Histological and histochemical findings in muscle spindles in dystrophia myotonica. J Neurol Sci 18:369–372, 1972.
20. Swash M: Muscle spindle pathology. In Mastaglia FL, Walton JN (eds): Skeletal Muscle Pathology. Edinburgh, Churchill Livingstone, 1982, pp 508–536.
21. Swash M, Schwartz MS: Normal muscle spindle morphology in myotonia congenita: The spindle abnormality in myotonic dystrophy is not due to myotonia alone. Clin Neuropathol 2:75–78, 1983.
22. Thomsen J: Tonische Krampfe in willkurlich beweglichen Muskeln infolge von ererbter psychischer Disposition (Ataxia muscularis?). Arch Psychiatr Nerv 6:702–718, 1876.
23. Becker PE: Myotonia Congenita and Syndromes Associated with Myotonia. Stuttgart, Thieme, 1977.
24. Kuhn E, Fiehn W, Seiler D, Schroeder JM: The autosomal recessive (Becker) form of myotonia congenita. Muscle Nerve 2:109–117, 1979.
25. Zellweger H, Pavone L, Biondi A, et al.: Autosomal recessive generalized myotonia. Muscle Nerve 3:176–180, 1980.
26. Sun SF, Streib EW: Autosomal recessive generalized myotonia. Muscle Nerve 6:143–148, 1983.
27. Crews J, Kaiser KK, Brooke MH: Muscle pathology of myotonia congenita. J Neurol Sci 28:449–457, 1976.
28. Eulenburg A: Uber eine familare, durch 6 Generationen verfolgbare Form congenitaler Paramyotonie. Neurol Zbl 5:265–272, 1886.
29. Riggs JE, Griggs RC, Moxley RT III: Acetazolamide-induced weakness in paramyotonia congenita. Ann Intern Med 86:169–173, 1977.

chapter 6

Periodic Paralyses and Glycogenoses

PERIODIC PARALYSES

Recurrent episodes of flaccid muscular weakness were recognized as a clinical entity long before the metabolic basis of the periodic paralyses was appreciated. The therapeutic value of potassium administration in the treatment of this condition was discovered empirically around the turn of the century. However, it was not until the 1930s that it was shown that these attacks of weakness were accompanied by a decrease in the serum potassium level.[1] Later, in the 1950s and 1960s, it was shown that other patients with periodic paralysis had elevated or normal potassium levels during their attacks.[2-4]

At the present time, three forms of periodic paralysis are generally recognized. These are designated as hypokalemic, hyperkalemic, and normokalemic, reflecting the levels of serum potassium that usually accompany spontaneous attacks. There is considerable overlap, especially between the hyperkalemic and normokalemic types. Brooke[5] found convincing evidence of hyperkalemic periodic paralysis in additional members of a kindred previously regarded by many authors as having normokalemic periodic paralysis.[2] Similarly, a patient previously reported by Meyers et al.[6] to have normokalemic periodic paralysis was restudied several years later by Chesson et al.[7] At that time, they found a complex mixture of attacks. Some were accompanied by hypokalemia, others were accompanied by hyperkalemia, while still others were accompanied by no change in the serum potassium level. The patient was able to distinguish these various types of attacks subjectively. Chesson et al.[7] designated this disorder as biphasic periodic paralysis. All forms of periodic paralysis are thought to be inherited as autosomal-dominant traits with a relatively high degree of penetrance. In addition, there are cases of hypokalemic periodic paralysis that are secondary to the use of various kaluretic agents or associated with other diseases.[8] The best known of these is the hypokalemic periodic paralysis associated with thyrotoxicosis. This disorder is found predominantly in individuals of Oriental extraction.

Familial hypokalemic periodic paralysis is the most common form of the periodic paralyses. The disorder affects males more frequently than females, even though it is an autosomal-dominant disease. A few cases, probably less than 5 percent, are apparently sporadic. The manifestations usually become evident during childhood or early adult life. At least initially, the paralytic episodes are relatively infrequent and typically occur at night. They may be precipitated by prior strenuous exercise or a high-carbohydrate meal. The episodes often last several hours to days. Although the attacks are rarely fatal, the patients may be nearly totally paralyzed with sparing of only the muscles of respiration and deglutition. Over the years, the attacks may recur with increasing frequency. In late adult life, the paralytic episodes may become less frequent but the disease may lead to permanent weakness.[9] The spontaneous attacks are characteristically accompanied by a fall in the level of the serum potassium. Attacks have been induced for diagnostic purposes by cautiously lowering the serum potassium by infusion of glucose and insulin.

Hyperkalemic periodic paralysis is also characterized by episodic weakness or muscular paralysis that begins in childhood. The sexes are affected equally. The attacks often occur during daytime and are usually briefer but more frequent than in patients with hypokalemic periodic paralysis. The attacks may be precipitated by exercise and exposure to cold. At least some of the patients display myotonia, especially of facial and hand muscles. The spontaneous attacks are typically accompanied by a rise in the serum potassium. Less often, the serum potassium remains unchanged and rarely, it may even decline.[9] Attacks have been induced for diagnostic purposes by the administration of potassium.

Normokalemic periodic paralysis shares many features in common with hyperkalemic periodic paralysis. The attacks begin early in life and the sexes are affected equally. The paralytic episodes may be precipitated by exercise and exposure to cold. Typically, the serum potassium level remains unchanged during the paralysis. In some patients, the attacks have been induced by the administration of potassium.

HISTOPATHOLOGY

All forms of the periodic paralyses may be associated with vacuolization of myofibers. In our experience, however, the vacuoles are most often seen in specimens from patients with hypokalemic periodic paralysis. The vacuoles are often more conspicuous when the biopsy specimens are obtained during a spontaneous or induced episode of paralysis. Specimens obtained between attacks, especially from individuals with disease of short duration, may show no diagnostic abnormalities. The vacuoles are most conspicuous in muscle specimens from individuals who have permanent myopathy as the result of long-standing disease with recurrent attacks of paralysis.[9] The vacuoles are often quite large and occupy the interior rather than the periphery of the affected myofibers (Fig. 6–1). Occasionally, they appear multiloculated, suggesting origin from the coalescence of smaller vacuoles. The vacuoles often appear "empty," with watery contents. Occasionally, they will contain PAS-positive granular material and rarely, histochemical stains will disclose the presence of calcium. By electron microscopy, the walls of the larger vacuoles can be shown to be in continuity with membranes of the T-tubules or with honeycomb arrays derived from the T-tubules (Fig. 6–2). Engel[10] has delineated four stages in the ultrastructural pathology of this disease: (1) the evolving vacuole, (2) the intermediate-stage vacuole, (3) the mature vacuole, and (4) the remodeling process. Initially, there are focal dilatations of the sarcoplasmic reticulum, abnormal arrays of T-tubules, and other forms of cytoplasmic degradation. Subsequent proliferations of membranes derived from the T-tubules entrap the foci of abnormal cytoplasmic organelles. The contents of these evolving vacuoles are then degraded by autophagy. Eventually, the mature vacuoles are in continuity with the extracellular spaces through the T-tubules. These ultrastructural findings explain the varied staining properties of the vacuolar contents observed by light microscopy. The vacuoles with contents undergoing autophagy appear

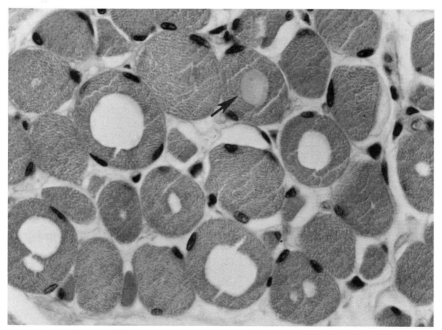

Figure 6–1. Paraffin-embedded section of muscle, stained with H&E, from a 17-year-old man with familial hypokalemic periodic paralysis. Note the numerous vacuoles of varying sizes. Although most appear empty, one *(arrow)* has finely granular contents. ×600.

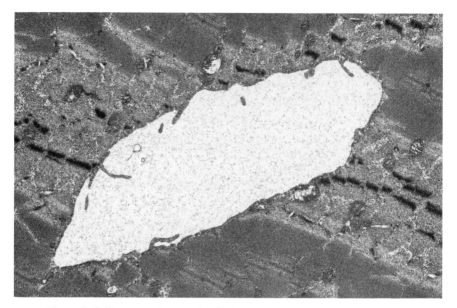

Figure 6-2. Electron micrograph of a large vacuole in a patient with hypokalemic periodic paralysis. The presence of incomplete septa reflects the origin from coalescence of smaller vacuoles. ×14,000.

PAS-positive while the mature vacuoles in continuity with the extracellular space appear "empty."

Tubular aggregates may be seen in muscle specimens from patients with hypokalemic periodic paralysis. They are, however, generally more conspicuous in specimens from patients with hyperkalemic or normokalemic periodic paralysis where they may comprise the major histopathologic findings (see below). Various nonspecific alterations also may be seen, especially by electron microscopy. The contractile elements may be in disarray resulting in foci of Z-disc streaming. Even target or at least targetoid fibers have been reported.[11] In some patients, ultrastructural examination has disclosed numerous concentric laminated bodies. These structures are hollow cylinders with walls composed of fibrillary laminae (Fig. 6–3). Each lamina appears to be formed by parallel circumferential fibrils and intersecting longitudinal fibrils. Similarly, filamentous bodies, relatively large compact skeins of tightly packed filaments (Fig. 6–4), may be present in some specimens. Although these structures are nonspecific and may be observed in other disorders, we have encountered them most often in the various forms of periodic paralyses. Occasionally, mitochondrial abnormalities, including the presence of intracristal paracrystalline arrays, may be encountered. Various abnormalities of the sarcoplasmic reticulum and T-tubules may be seen and may be early stages in the evolution of the vacuoles. Lipofuscin may be increased. This is probably the end-stage of the autophagic activity following remodeling of the vacuoles.

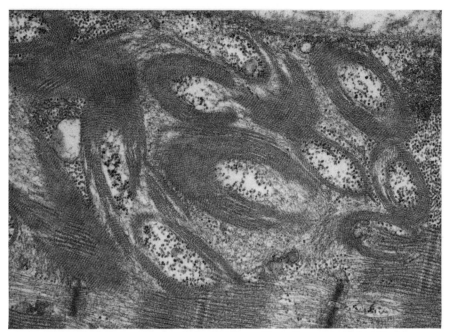

Figure 6-3. Concentric laminated bodies with walls composed of fibrillary laminae are among the nonspecific structures that may be seen by electron microscopy in biopsy specimens from patients with hypokalemic periodic paralysis. ×37,500.

Muscle specimens from patients with hypokalemic periodic paralysis in association with hyperthyroidism,[12,13] hyperaldosteronism,[14] and secondary to the use of various kaluretic agents show changes that are similar to but generally milder than seen with the familial form of the disease. The special precipitating circumstances or underlying diseases are not evident from examination of the muscle specimens.

Often the most striking abnormality in specimens from patients with hyperkalemic or normokalemic periodic paralysis is the presence of tubular aggregates. In sections stained with H&E, these appear as abnormal basophilic deposits in the interior or at the periphery of the affected myofibers. The aggregates are further characterized by their intense red staining with the modified trichrome procedure (Fig. 6–5) and dark blue staining with the NADH–TR reaction. They can be distinguished from mitochondrial deposits by their failure to stain with the SDH reaction. They are found predominantly but not exclusively in type II myofibers. Tubular aggregates have a granular appearance in epoxy-embedded sections (Fig. 6–6). By electron microscopy they appear as randomly oriented fascicles of parallel tubules (Fig. 6–7). The individual tubules measure 60 to 90 nm in diameter and have smooth osmiophilic walls. The tubules are generally closely aggregated and are occasionally fused, giving

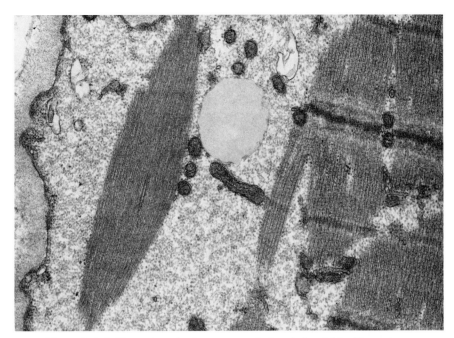

Figure 6-4. A filamentous body, composed of a skein of thin filaments *(left of center)* is another nonspecific structure that may be seen by electron microscopy. ×38,000

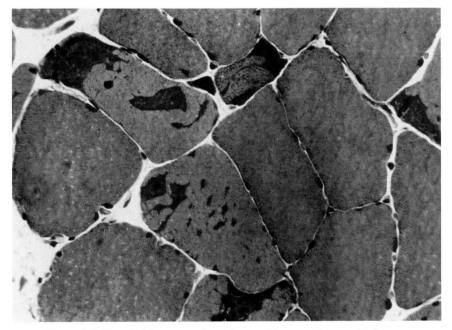

Figure 6-5. Muscle biopsy specimen from a 20-year-old man with hyperkalemic periodic paralysis. Although vacuoles are not evident, there are prominent red-staining tubular aggregates at the periphery and in the interior of several myofibers. Trichrome, ×420.

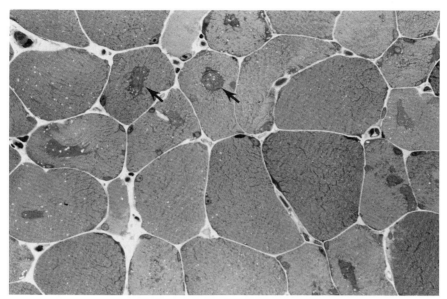

Figure 6-6. The tubular aggregates *(arrows)* have a granular appearance when seen in epoxy-embedded sections. Toluidine blue, ×420.

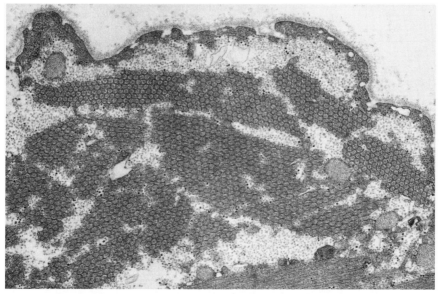

Figure 6-7. Electron micrograph showing a tubular aggregate in cross-section. ×30,000

rise to dumbbell, trefoil, or even more complex cross-sectional profiles. The lumina of the tubules often contain coaxial inner tubules, rodlets, or granular material. Often they are coextensive with and appear to arise from the terminal cisterns of the sarcoplasmic reticulum (Fig. 6–8). Less often, another type of tubule is encountered. These tubules are less closely aggregated and are further characterized by the presence of longitudinally oriented filaments applied to their exterior surface. Whether these striated tubules are also derived from the sarcoplasmic reticulum has not been established.

TUBULAR AGGREGATE MYOPATHIES

As indicated, tubular aggregates are especially abundant in hyperkalemic and normokalemic period paralysis. Occasionally they have been described in other conditions, such as porphyria, drug intoxication,[15] alcoholic myopathy,[16] myotonic dystrophy, and other myotonias.[17] They also comprise the major morphologic abnormality in individuals with the so-called "tubular aggregate" myopathies.[18–21] These patients generally have exercise-induced cramps and mild weakness but no myoglobinuria. Both familial and sporadic cases have been reported. Morphologic studies have revealed varying numbers of tubular aggregates, predominantly in type II myofibers (Figs. 6–9 and 6–10). Some of the specimens have also shown abundant cytoplasmic bodies and increased var-

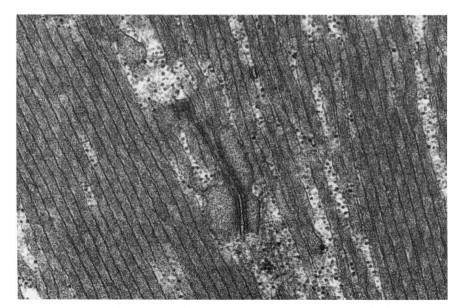

Figure 6–8. Electron micrograph of a tubular aggregate in longitudinal section. The tubules are in continuity with dilated terminal cisterns of the sarcoplasmic reticulum. ×60,000.

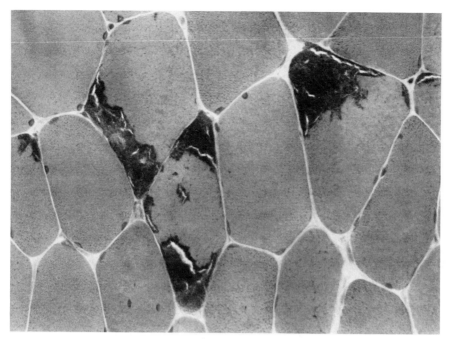

Figure 6-9. Tubular aggregate myopathy. This 36-year-old man complained of decreased exercise tolerance and occasional muscular aches. There was no evidence of periodic paralysis. The tubular aggregates stained dark red with the trichrome procedure. ×430.

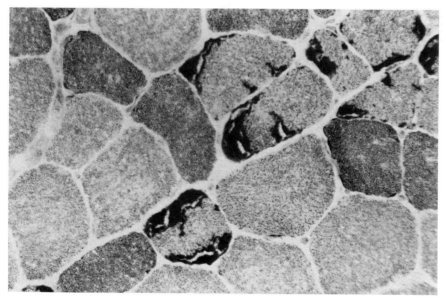

Figure 6-10. Tubular aggregate myopathy. The tubular aggregates stained dark blue with the NADH–TR reaction. They are found predominantly in the lighter-staining type II myofibers. NADH–TR, ×410.

iation in myofiber size, due mainly to type II atrophy. The precise nature of this condition or group of conditions is unknown.

GLYCOGEN AND THE GLYCOGENOSES

Glycogen in Normal Muscle

Carbohydrates and lipids are metabolized by skeletal muscle in different proportions depending upon the type and duration of muscular activity. At rest, skeletal muscle utilizes free fatty acids predominantly. During sudden intense exercise, the intracellular stores of glycogen are the major source of energy after preformed stores of high-energy phosphates are exhausted. With prolonged exercise, fatty acids are mobilized and again become the major metabolic substrate. Several of the glycogenoses are manifested predominantly during periods of intense energy demand, reflecting the normal variations in substrate utilization.

The overall glycogen content of normal skeletal muscle is relatively constant since glycogen itself inhibits glycogen synthesis and promotes phosphorolysis.[22] By histochemical techniques, apparent differences in glycogen content can be demonstrated among the various fiber types. In frozen sections stained with the PAS techniques, the type II myofibers, especially the type IIB myofibers are stained more intensely. These staining differences are not sufficiently striking or consistently reproducible to be used reliably for fiber typing. Paradoxically, biochemical studies on isolated myofibers have shown essentially the same glycogen content in both type I and type II myofibers.[23] A lack of staining, however, presumably reflecting the absence of glycogen, is readily evident in myofibers undergoing necrosis. In paraffin-embedded sections, the various fiber types show less conspicuous differences in their staining with the PAS reactions.

By electron microscopy, glycogen in skeletal muscle normally appears as so-called beta particles. These are individual, moderately osmiophilic granules that generally range from 15 to 35 nm in diameter. The glycogen granules are most numerous at the periphery of the myofiber within the subsarcolemmal space adjacent to the nuclei, and within the intermyofibrillar spaces. The larger, more complex aggregates of glycogen, the so-called alpha rosettes, are not seen in skeletal muscle. During processing for electron microscopy, glycogen tends to be leached out of muscle subjected to prolonged block staining with uranyl magnesium acetate.[24] Therefore, we occasionally process additional tissue with the block staining step omitted when detailed evaluation of the glycogen content is desired. An apparent increase in the glycogen content must be interpreted with caution since an increase in the number of glycogen granules is encountered as a nonspecific response in many pathologic processes. As with most metabolic diseases, the definitive diagnosis of a glycogenosis depends on biochemical characterization of the stored material and demonstration of corresponding enzyme deficiency. Currently there are at least eight glycogenoses for which enzyme deficiencies have been described. Several of these directly involve skeletal muscle and have morphologically discernible abnormalities (Table 6–1).

Type II Glycogenoses

The type II glycogenoses are associated with a deficiency in acid maltase activity. This is a lysosomal enzyme that cleaves 1–4- and 1–6-alpha-glycosidic linkages. Since this hydrolytic lysosomal enzyme is not in the main degradative or synthetic pathways for glycogen, some authors have suggested that the enzyme deficiency is an epiphenomenon rather than the basic metabolic defect in these disorders.[25] Nevertheless, the demonstration of a deficiency in acid maltase activity is generally considered satisfactory biochemical confirmation for these diseases.

Type II glycogenosis occurs in two well characterized but very dissimilar forms, the infantile form otherwise known as Pompe's disease and the so-called adult form. In addition, there is a less well-delineated juvenile form. Infants with Pompe's disease have hypotonia, weak but firm muscles, macroglossia, cardiomegaly, congestive heart failure, and hepatomegaly. The latter is at least in part due to the congestive heart failure. The disease is inexorably progressive and the children die within 1 or 2 years. Abnormal storage of glycogen occurs

TABLE 6-1. GLYCOGENOSES

Type II glycogenosis (Pompe's disease)	Severely vacuolated myofibers Scattered deposits of basophilic mucopolysaccharide Increased acid phosphatase activity
Type II glycogenosis (AAMD)	Few to many vacuolated fibers Granules that are red with the trichrome stain Increased acid phosphatase activity Ring fibers
Lysosomal glycogen storage disease with normal acid maltase activity	Numerous vacuolated fibers with amphophilic contents Granules that are red with the trichrome stain Increased acid phosphatase activity
Type III glycogenosis	Moderate to severely vacuolated fibers Ring fibers
Type IV glycogenosis	Scattered aggregates of polyglucosan bodies
Type V glycogenosis	Few to many scattered subsarcolemmal vacuoles No myophosphorylase activity
Type VII glycogenosis	Subsarcolemmal vacuoles Rare polyglucosan bodies Normal myophosphorylase activity

in many organs including the central nervous system, heart, liver, and skeletal muscles. The intramuscular storage of glycogen is more severe in Pompe's disease than in the other glycogenoses. Nevertheless, there is considerable variation in the degree of involvement from muscle to muscle.

Frozen sections from affected muscles generally disclose severe vacuolation of the myofibers. With H&E, the vacuoles appear to be empty or to contain finely granular material. The contents are PAS-positive and are extensively digested with diastase, reflecting the presence of glycogen. In addition, there may be deposits of basophilic material that is PAS-positive but resistant to diastase digestion. This latter material is thought to be a mucopolysaccharide.[26,27] The source of this material and its relation to the massive accumulation of glycogen is unclear. Stains for acid phosphatase activity are strongly positive in many of the vacuoles, reflecting the increased lysosomal activity secondary to the acid maltase deficiency. At least some specimens also have vacuoles containing neutral lipids that are stainable with oil red O.[28]

Paraffin-embedded sections of muscle also demonstrate extensive vacuolation of myofibers (Fig. 6–11). With H&E, most of the vacuoles appear to be empty but some contain amorphous basophilic mucopolysaccharide. The deposits of basophilic material are more conspicuous when the tissue has been fixed in a strongly acid fixative like SUSA solution (Fig. 6–12). Periodic acid-Schiff-positive material may be evident at the edges of otherwise empty vacuoles and within the myofibers between vacuoles.

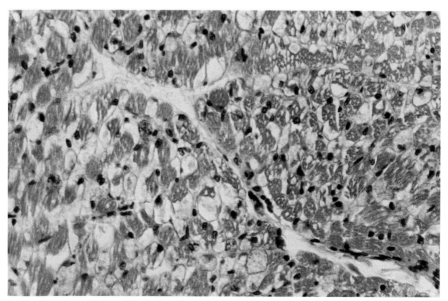

Figure 6–11. Paraffin-embedded section of a muscle biopsy specimen from a 3½-month-old boy with Pompe's disease. Note the extensive vacuolation of the myofibers. H&E, ×410.

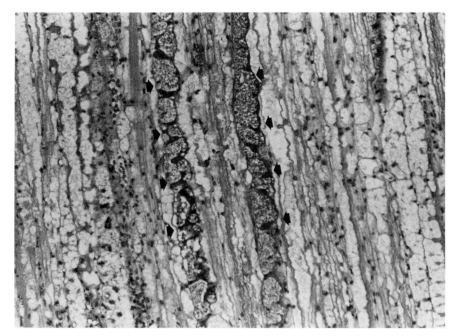

Figure 6-12. Muscle obtained at autopsy from a 7-month-old boy with Pompe's disease. The basophilic granular mucopolysaccharide *(arrows)* is readily seen in this paraffin-embedded section of tissue that had been fixed in SUSA solution. H&E, ×180.

By electron microscopy, muscle specimens from children with Pompe's disease show massive accumulation of glycogen granules. These are found beneath the sarcolemma and between the myofibrils. The individual myofibrils often appear abnormally thin or atrophic when the myofiber is massively distended by the glycogen accumulation. Much of the abnormal glycogen is free in the sarcoplasm with only a portion confined within lysosomal membranes. The glycogen granules within the lysosomes often show a different degree of osmiophilia and may appear either lighter or darker than the surrounding free glycogen. At least some of the intralysosomal glycogen accumulates because of the lysosomal acid maltase deficiency. The associated myofiber damage has been attributed to leakage of acidic hydrolases from the abnormally distended lysosomes. Whether the free glycogen deposits result from rupture of distended lysosomes or arise through some other mechanism is uncertain. Furthermore, it seems paradoxical that free glycogen should accumulate abnormally in the presence of normal phosphorylase activity.

The childhood and adult forms of acid maltase deficiency are manifested predominantly as myopathies. The childhood form becomes evident early in life with delayed development, weakness of the proximal limb muscles and respiratory muscles, and occasionally hypertrophy of the calves. Although the disease progresses slowly, most of the patients die by the end of the second decade of life as the result of respiratory complications. As the name suggests, the adult form presents in adulthood. The patients have slowly progressive muscular weakness, and initially are often thought to have limb girdle dystrophy or a chronic inflammatory myopathy.[29,30] Acid maltase deficiency should be considered in such patients, especially when myotonic discharges are demonstrated by electrophysiologic studies.[31] Some of the patients have respiratory failure and die from the involvement of the intercostal muscles and diaphragm.[32] In contrast to the infantile form, the heart and liver are generally uninvolved and the skeletal muscles accumulate far less glycogen. In some muscles, the glycogen content may even be within the normal range.

Both frozen and paraffin-embedded sections reveal vacuoles in scattered myofibers (Figs. 6–13 and 6–14). Clinically involved muscles contain a higher proportion of vacuolated fibers than uninvolved muscles.[33] Nevertheless, the vacuolation is much less severe and less extensive than in the infantile form of the disease. The type I myofibers are generally more prominently affected, although in at least one childhood case preferential involvement of the type II myofibers was reported.[34] The vacuolar contents are PAS-positive and partially diastase digestible, reflecting their glycogen content. Deposits of basophilic mucopolysaccharide may be seen in the childhood cases but are inconspicuous or absent in the adult cases. Increased acid phosphatase activity is demonstrable in the vacuoles and in scattered foci within nonvacuolated myofibers (Fig. 6–

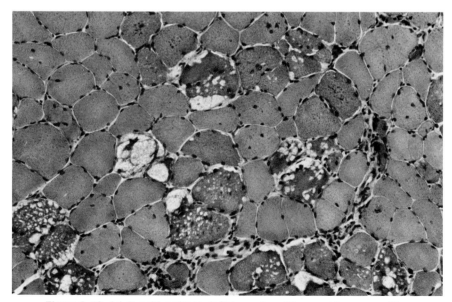

Figure 6-13. Adult acid maltase deficiency in a 31-year-old woman with a 10-year history of progressive proximal muscular weakness. Note the scattered vacuolated myofibers. H&E, × 180.

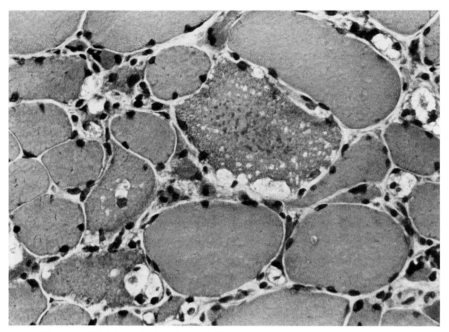

Figure 6-14. Adult acid maltase deficiency in a 50-year-old woman with a 10-year history of proximal weakness first manifested by difficulty climbing stairs. The vacuoles are of varying size and some are accompanied by small eosinophilic granules. H&E, ×430.

15). There is a similar increase in esterase activity as demonstrated with the nonspecific esterase reaction. Abnormal deposits of lipid droplets also have been reported in some of the adult cases.[30]

Karpati et al.[35] reported scattered small angular myofibers of both major fiber types and fiber-type grouping in an adult patient with acid maltase deficiency. On the basis of these morphologic features of neurogenic atrophy and reinnervation and supportive electromyographic findings, the authors suggested that motor neuron involvement may contribute to the muscle weakness and wasting in these patients. However, autopsy studies on a childhood patient and an adult patient[34,36] have failed to show glycogen storage within the central nervous system, including spinal motor neurons.

Electron microscopic studies of muscle specimens from patients with the childhood and adult forms of acid maltase deficiency disclose multiple, focal deposits of glycogen. Much of the glycogen is free in the sarcoplasm, especially beneath the sarcolemma and within the intermyofibrillar spaces. Some of the glycogen is membrane bound. Often the membrane-bound glycogen is accompanied by granular osmiophilic and lamellar material (Fig. 6–16). These aggregates resemble autophagic vacuoles and residual bodies. Rarely, enlarged mitochondria with intracristal paracrystalline arrays have been reported.[37] We

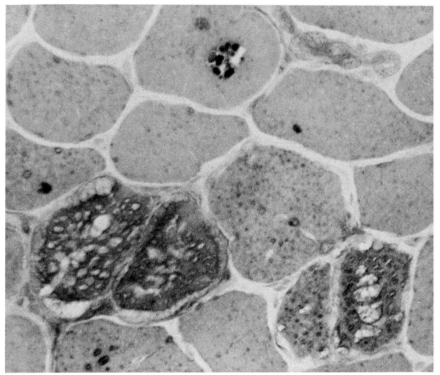

Figure 6-15. Increased acid phosphatase activity can be demonstrated around the vacuoles and in scattered nonvacuolated myofibers. ×410.

have also encountered filamentous bodies in a case of adult acid maltase deficiency.

The biochemical basis for the varied clinical and morphologic expressions of acid maltase deficiency in the infantile, childhood, and adult forms have been the subject of extensive investigation. Current hypotheses implicate selective involvement of acid maltase isoenzymes,[38] concurrent involvement of neutral maltase in the infantile form,[39] and higher residual acid maltase activity in the childhood and adult forms.[40,41] Furthermore, the biochemical basis for the selective involvement of the skeletal muscles in the presence of systemic acid maltase deficiency in the adult form of the disease remains unresolved.[41] There is at least one report of both the infantile and adult forms of acid maltase deficiency occurring in different members of a single family.[42]

Lysosomal Glycogen Storage Disease with Normal Acid Maltase Activity

Morphologic correlation between intralysosomal glycogen accumulation and acid maltase deficiency has been further complicated by cases recently reported by Danon et al.[43] and Riggs et al.[44] Although occasional membrane-bound de-

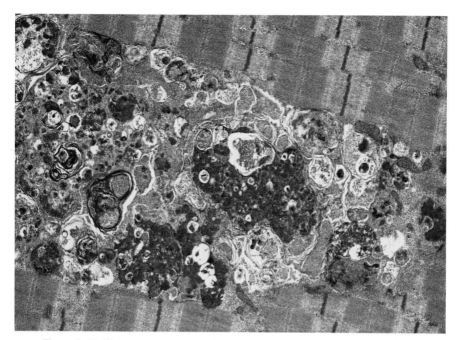

Figure 6-16. Electron micrograph of muscle biopsy specimen from a 48-year-old man with adult acid maltase deficiency. Free and membrane-bound glycogen particles are accompanied by osmiophilic, finely granular, and lamellar material. The latter components correspond to the eosinophilic granular material seen by light microscopy. × 13,150.

posits of glycogen may develop as a nonspecific response in the presence of abundant free glycogen, numerous lysosomes harboring glycogen were generally considered to be the morphologic hallmark of acid maltase deficiency. The cases reported by these authors appear to delineate another form of glycogenosis, with prominent intralysosomal glycogen storage in the presence of normal acid maltase activity. The patients reported by Danon et al.[43] were two unrelated teenage boys who had proximal muscle weakness, hypertrophic cardiomyopathy, and mental retardation. One also had hepatomegaly. The patients reported by Riggs et al.[44] were teenage brothers. These patients also had proximal muscle weakness, hypertrophic cardiomyopathy, and probable intellectual impairment. To date, the number of reported cases is insufficient to determine the pattern of inheritance.

The histochemical studies on the skeletal muscle specimens from these cases of lysosomal glycogen storage disease revealed a vacuolar myopathy. In frozen sections, stained with H&E, the vacuoles appeared to be empty or to contain fine granular basophilic material. Some of this material stained red with the modified trichrome technique (Fig. 6–17) and was at least partially PAS-positive. Many of the vacuoles showed increased acid phosphatase and

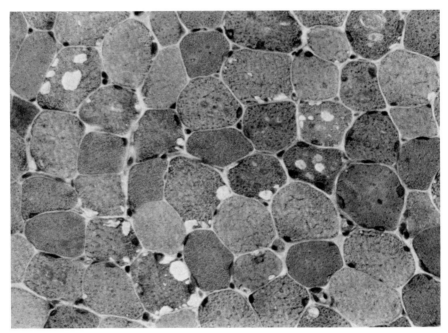

Figure 6-17. Lysosomal glycogen storage disease with normal acid maltase activity. This muscle biopsy specimen is from a 14-year-old boy, one of the two brothers reported by Riggs et al.[44] The vacuoles contain finely granular material and are found in fibers of both types but predominantly in type I myofibers. Trichrome, ×440.

nonspecific esterase activity. Both fiber types were affected, however, vacuolation was more prominent in type I myofibers.

By electron microscopy, the subsarcolemmal and intermyofibrillar spaces contained free glycogen granules and fine fibrillar material. The free glycogen was somewhat less abundant than usually seen in cases of adult acid maltase deficiency. The membrane-bound glycogen was contained in numerous small residual bodies along with osmiophilic lamellar and granular material.

Biochemical studies demonstrated a slight but significant increase in muscle glycogen content and, in the cases reported by Riggs et al.,[44] a slight but probably nonspecific increase in acid maltase activity. The biochemical basis for this disorder has not yet been elucidated. These cases illustrate the limitations of morphology with regard to metabolic diseases and emphasize the need for biochemical evaluation in order to establish a definitive diagnosis.

Type III Glycogenosis

Type III glycogenosis is due to deficient activity of one or both components of the debranching enzyme complex. This includes both an oligotransferase that moves a three-carbon oligosaccharide, and the actual debranching activity by amylo-1,6-glucosidase. Some authors regard the disease to be relatively common, possibly the most common of the glycogenoses.[25,38,45] Various patterns of clinical disease have been described. Most often, the disease is encountered as a mild disorder of childhood dominated by hepatomegaly and delayed development. These children may have increased susceptibility to infections and occasional seizures. Some show a preference for starchy foods. In a few of the affected children, the disease is also manifested by muscular weakness, hypotonia, and atrophy.[46] Because of their inability to properly catabolize glycogen, clinical laboratory studies will show mild fasting hypoglycemia, ketonuria, and hyperlipidemia. Many of these children show marked improvement or even total remission of symptoms during adolescence.

Morphologic studies on muscle biopsy specimens from childhood cases of type III glycogenosis are rather limited. Pellissier et al.[46] described their findings in a biopsy specimen from the rectus abdominis muscle of a 4-year-old girl. The specimen disclosed increased variation in myofiber size, type I myofiber predominance, and scattered vacuolated myofibers. The vacuoles were subsarcolemmal and internal in location and involved fibers of both major fiber types. The vacuolar contents were PAS-positive, and by electron microscopy they appeared as large collections of glycogen granules. In addition to the glycogen storage, the authors also described type I myofiber predominance and myofibrillar alterations that they interpreted as multicore structures. The authors suggested that the latter structures were unrelated to the glycogenosis and constituted evidence of coexistent multicore disease. Alternatively, these findings could be interpreted as evidence of neurogenic involvement as part of the glycogen storage disorder (see below).

Adults with type III glycogenosis may be asymptomatic or have a late-onset myopathy. The latter patients have varying degrees of exercise intolerance, proximal muscular weakness, and distal muscular wasting.[47-49] In some of the adults, hepatomegaly and muscular symptoms persist from childhood. Because of the distal wasting, fasciculations, and fibrillations, several of these patients have been diagnosed initially as having motor neuron disease.[47-49]

Histologic studies of muscle biopsy specimens from adults with type III glycogenosis have disclosed multiple vacuoles in myofibers of both major fiber types. The vacuolation may be extensive and occur throughout the whole muscle fiber (Fig. 6-18) or may be predominantly subsarcolemmal in location. The vacuolar contents are PAS-positive and at least partially digestible with diastase. Ring fibers were a conspicuous feature in several of the adult cases reported by DiMauro et al.[48] and were present along with targetoid fibers in the case reported by Brunberg et al.[47] Electron microscopy discloses numerous free glycogen granules beneath the sarcolemma and to a lesser extent, within intermyofibrillar spaces (Fig. 6-19). Where especially abundant, some of the glycogen granules may be surrounded by membranes (Fig. 6-20). As previously mentioned, occasional membrane-bound deposits of glycogen can occur as a nonspecific response to the presence of abundant intracytoplasmic glycogen, regardless of the cause.

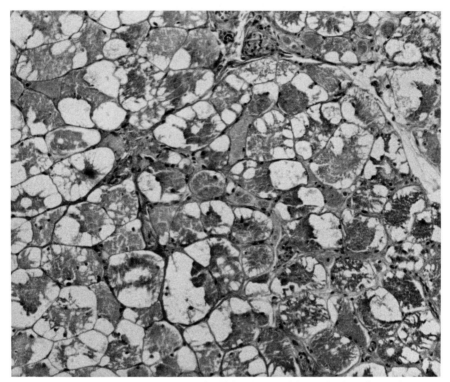

Figure 6-18. Type III glycogenosis. This 43-year-old man had an 8-month history of muscular weakness and atrophy of distal arm and hand muscles. Numerous large vacuoles are seen in this paraffin-embedded section of a SUSA-fixed muscle biopsy specimen. Trichrome, × 200.

Type IV Glycogenosis

Type IV glycogenosis is associated with a deficiency in the activity of the brancher enzyme, alpha-1,4-glucan: alpha-1,4-glucan, 6-glycosyl transferase.[45] Many tissues are affected and contain deposits of an abnormal carbohydrate with relatively few branch points. This abnormal polysaccharide is biochemically similar to amylopectin.[50] Some of the patients come to medical attention early in life as "floppy infants."[51] This aspect of their illness is rapidly overshadowed, however, by the development of hepatic dysfunction and cirrhosis.[52,53] Death generally occurs within the first few years of life from hepatic failure or occasionally, cardiac involvement.

Histologic examination of the liver reveals a finely nodular cirrhosis with pseudonodules delineated by thin fibrous septa. The hepatocytes contain prominent deposits of finely granular adventitious material. This material is faintly basophilic with H&E, strongly PAS-positive, and brown with Lugol's iodine.[52,53] By electron microscopy, the intrahepatic carbohydrate deposits ap-

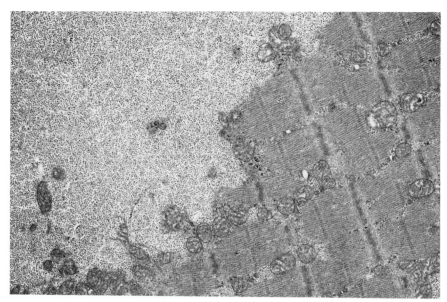

Figure 6-19. Type III glycogenosis. Electron micrograph showing large collection of free glycogen granules. ×20,000.

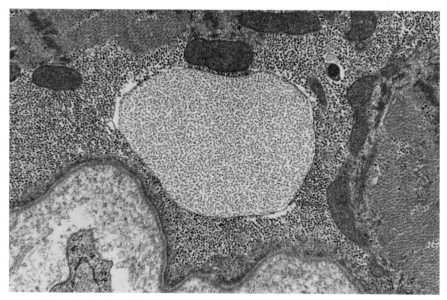

Figure 6-20. Type III glycogenosis. Electron micrograph showing one of the rare membrane-bound collections of glycogen granules. ×30,000.

pear to consist of glycogen in the form of alpha rosettes and beta particles and an abnormal fibrillar polysaccharide. Examination of the central nervous system has disclosed deposits of abnormal carbohydrate in the form of minute spheroids within the cytoplasm of astrocytes.[52,54] These are most numerous in the subpial region and about blood vessels and resemble small corpora amylacea. They have staining properties that are similar to the intrahepatic deposits. By electron microscopy, they appear as compact masses of branched osmiophilic fibrils.

Abnormal deposits of polysaccharide have been described in the skeletal muscles in about half of the reported cases of type IV glycogenosis.[54,55] The deposits are not uniformly distributed, and in some patients they have been most abundant in the tongue and diaphragm. The individual deposits consist of small collections of spheroidal or polyhedral granules (Fig. 6–21) that are often located at the periphery of the affected myofibers. The granules stain blue with H&E, trichrome, and alcian blue, red with Best carmine, and black with methenamine silver. They are strongly PAS-positive (Fig. 6–22). The carbohydrate deposits are hydrolyzed by pectinase but are only minimally affected by alpha or beta amylases. By electron microscopy, the deposits appear as unbounded aggregates of branched osmiophilic fibrils and osmiophilic granular

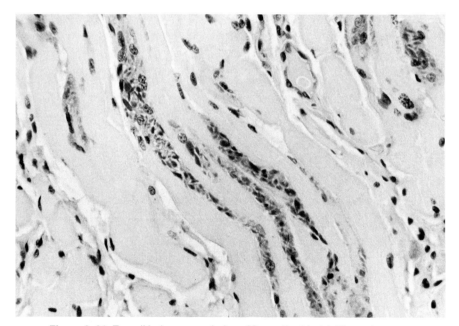

Figure 6–21. Type IV glycogenosis in a 28-month-old girl. The polysaccharide deposits have a polyhedral configuration and are distributed unevenly among the myofibers in this paraffin-embedded section. The muscle was obtained at the time of autopsy and fixed in SUSA solution. PAS, × 430.

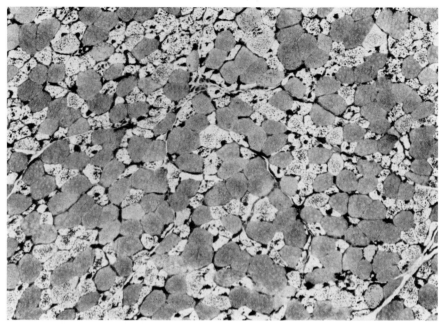

Figure 6-22. Type IV glycogenosis in an 8-year-old girl who initially presented with congestive heart failure. This rectus abdominis muscle biopsy specimen displays numerous deposits of abnormal PAS-positive polysaccharide, predominantly in atrophic myofibers. PAS, × 175. *(Case provided by Roger E. Riepe, M.D., Wesley Medical Center, Wichita, Kansas.)*

material (Figs. 6–23 and 6–24). The deposits in the myocardium are similar to those in skeletal muscle.

Ultrastructurally, and to a lesser extent histochemically, the carbohydrate deposits in type IV glycogenosis are remarkably similar to Lafora bodies, corpora amylacea, and basophilic degeneration of the myocardium. Whether these diverse carbohydrate deposits have a similar pathogenesis remains speculative.

Type V Glycogenosis

Type V glycogenosis, otherwise known as McArdle's disease, results from a deficiency of myophosphorylase activity. Myophosphorylase cleaves 1,4-alpha-glucosidic linkages, releasing glucose moieties from glycogen chains. The enzymatic deficiency may result from the absence of the enzyme or from the presence of an aberrant inactive form of the enzyme.[56,57] When the myophosphorylase activity is deficient, intramuscular glycogen cannot be utilized as a source of glucose for anaerobic glycolysis. Thus the enzyme deficiency is manifested predominantly during brief periods of high energy demand. The failure of venous lactate to increase during ischemic exercise reflects the reduced utilization of anaerobic glycolysis. This laboratory finding is character-

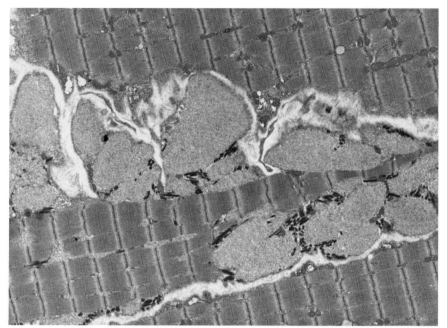

Figure 6-23. Type IV glycogenosis. This electron micrograph shows the abnormal polysaccharide deposits at the periphery of the myofiber. × 15,200. *(Case provided by Roger E. Riepe, M.D., Wesley Medical Center, Wichita, Kansas.)*

istic but not pathognomonic of myophosphorylase deficiency, since deficient lactate production can also be seen with type VI and type VII glycogenoses.

Several different patterns of clinical manifestations have now been described. Most patients with type V glycogenosis have a history of exercise intolerance dating back to childhood or adolescence. Initially, strenuous exercise produces muscle pain, stiffness, and fatigue. These manifestations may be relieved by a period of rest. Later in adulthood, overexertion may produce muscle cramps and episodes of rhabdomyolysis with myoglobinuria or even renal failure.[8,25] About one third of these patients eventually develop persistent mild proximal weakness.[25] Some patients with type V glycogenosis do not experience the initial manifestations of their disease until later in adult life. One woman who had been physically active and previously free of muscle symptoms, abruptly developed muscle cramps, stiffness, and swelling accompanied by myoglobinuria at the age of 60.[57] Other adults with this disease have presented as a late-onset myopathy with progressive weakness but no cramps or myoglobinuria.[58] There are also atypical cases that become manifest very early in life. A fatal infantile form of myophosphorylase deficiency was delineated in two female infants who developed rapidly progressive weakness at about 1 month of age and died of respiratory failure.[59,60] An early childhood form has

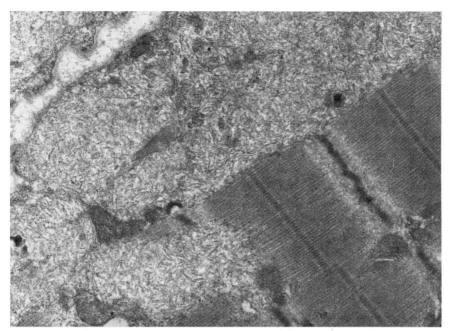

Figure 6-24. Type IV glycogenosis. This high-magnification electron micrograph shows the fibrillar nature of the abnormal polysaccharide. ×76,000. *(Case provided by Roger E. Riepe, M.D., Wesley Medical Center, Wichita, Kansas.)*

been described in a 4-year-old boy with proximal muscle weakness and an abnormal gait resembling Duchenne muscular dystrophy.[61]

Frozen sections, and less consistently, paraffin-embedded sections of skeletal muscle from adults with McArdle's disease will often disclose abnormal deposits of glycogen. The deposits usually appear as small subsarcolemmal vacuoles or blebs (Fig. 6-25). Other smaller deposits also may be seen as minute vacuoles within the interior of the myofibers. The vacuolar contents are PAS-positive and are at least partially digestible with diastase. In some patients, virtually no vacuoles are evident by light microscopy.

A diagnosis of McArdle's disease usually can be established by the histochemical evaluation of myophosphorylase activity. This procedure employs iodine to demonstrate elongation of glycogen chains by glucose-1-phosphate in the presence of myophosphorylase. Thus the histochemical assay reaction is the opposite of the reaction normally catalyzed by myophosphorylase in vivo. Normally type II myofibers stain more intensely than type I myofibers, however in specimens from patients with McArdle's disease, there is no staining among intact myofibers of either type (Fig. 6-26). Regenerating myofibers following rhabdomyolysis, and smooth muscle fibers in vessel walls will be stained. It is important to monitor the histochemical procedure with a control speci-

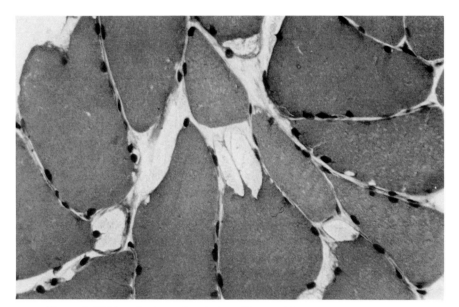

Figure 6-25. Type V glycogenosis in a 37-year-old woman. Note the small subsarcolemmal vacuoles. H&E, ×440.

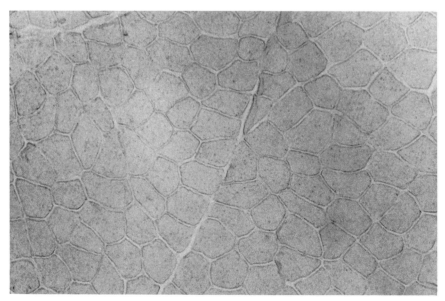

Figure 6-26. Type V glycogenosis in a 42-year-old man. Note the virtual absence of staining with the myophosphorylase technique. ×180.

men. Muscle from a patient suspected of having McArdle's disease and the control subject can be compared readily by having sections from both mounted on a single slide (Fig. 6–27). Nevertheless, patients with partial myophosphorylase deficiency may escape detection by the usual histochemical procedure since as little as 10 percent of normal myophosphorylase activity will result in staining.[57,58] The staining of regenerating myofibers has been attributed to the presence of an isoenzyme, the so-called "fetal myophosphorylase."[59] Similarly, the absence of cardiac involvement in McArdle's disease has been attributed to the presence of other isoenzymes.[60]

Electron microscopy of skeletal muscle specimens from patients with McArdle's disease reveals abnormal deposits of glycogen granules beneath the sarcolemma and to a lesser extent, within the intermyofibrillar spaces.[62] The glycogen granules appear as the usual beta particles. Occasionally, when especially abundant, some of the glycogen is found within membrane-bound spaces, i.e., intralysosomal. A comparative study of muscle ultrastructure before and after ischemic exercise disclosed only minimal changes such as dilatation of the sarcoplasmic reticulum and degeneration of mitochondria following the exercise.[63]

Type VII Glycogenosis

Type VII glycogenosis or Tarui's disease is a rare disorder of carbohydrate metabolism that results from a partial deficiency of muscle phosphofructo-kinase activity.[63] This enzyme catalyzes the conversion of fructose-6-phosphate

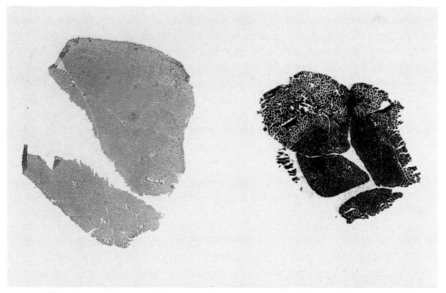

Figure 6-27. Sections from a patient with McArdle's disease *(left)* and from a normal control subject *(right)* mounted together and stained simultaneously. Myophosphorylase, × 1.75.

to fructose-1,6-diphosphate and is one of the main rate-limiting steps of glycolysis. When phosphofructokinase activity is deficient, neither glucose nor glycogen can be utilized effectively as a source of energy. As in McArdle's disease, the block in anaerobic glycolysis is reflected by failure of ischemic exercise to elevate venous lactate. At least some cases of type VII glycogenosis will, however, show enhanced venous lactate production following administration of glucagon.[64] Another effect of the phosphofructokinase deficiency is elevation of glucose-6-phosphate. This activates glycogen synthetase leading to still more glycogen accumulation.

Type VII glycogenosis may be manifested in several different ways. Most of the patients have a disorder that is similar to McArdle's disease. Beginning in childhood, the patients display exercise intolerance, cramps, and occasionally myoglobinuria.[25,65] Most also have mild hemolytic anemia due to an associated deficiency of erythrocyte phosphofructokinase activity. Other adults have had a myopathy with progressive weakness but no cramps or episodes of myoglobinuria.[66] Recently, cases involving infants also have been described. These children have weakness and congenital fixation of joints.[67]

Frozen and paraffin-embedded sections of muscle from patients with type VII glycogenosis usually show scattered subsarcolemmal and intermyofibrillar deposits of glycogen. The deposits are PAS-positive and are at least partially digestible with diastase. Electron microscopy demonstrates morphologically normal beta glycogen particles. Scattered degenerating and regenerating myofibers may be encountered if the patient has had a recent episode of rhabdomyolysis and myoglobinuria. These morphologic features are virtually identical to those seen in cases of McArdle's disease. A presumptive diagnosis of type VII glycogenosis can be established in some of these patients with typical clinical findings and a vacuolar myopathy by the histochemical demonstration of normal myophosphorylase activity. Although phosphofructokinase activity can be evaluated histochemically,[68] this procedure is often not included in the routine evaluation of muscle biopsy specimens.

Unfortunately, this approach will not detect all cases of type VII glycogenosis. Frozen sections from the infants with this disorder showed variation in myofiber size with numerous small fibers but no vacuolation or abnormal deposits of PAS-positive material.[67] However, epoxy-embedded sections revealed small, crescent-shaped subsarcolemmal deposits in about 20 percent of the myofibers. Electron microscopy disclosed excessive subsarcolemmal and intermyofibrillar accumulations of free glycogen granules. Rare deposits were membrane-bound.

Recently, an additional morphologic feature has been reported in muscle biopsy specimens from some patients with phosphofructokinase deficiency.[66,69] Distinctive polyglucosan inclusions were found individually and in small groups in 2 to 10 percent of the myofibers. Both major fiber types were similarly affected. The inclusions were stained blue–gray with H&E, red with Best carmine, and black with methenamine silver. They were PAS-positive and stained brown with iodine. The polyglucosan bodies resisted digestion with diastase, beta amylase, and pectinase. They were, however, partially or completely removed with alpha and gamma amylases. By electron microscopy, the inclusions appeared to be composed of compact masses of filaments, 6 to 8 nm in diameter. Tubular profiles, mitochondria, and occasional dense bodies were admixed among the filaments. These polyglucosan bodies had many morphologic, histochemical, and ultrastructural features in common with the polysaccharide deposits found in type IV glycogenosis. It has been suggested that the polyglucosan bodies encountered in type VII glycogenosis resulted from activation of glycogen synthetase by the elevated levels of glucose-6-phosphate.[69]

We have recently studied a child with recurrent hemolysis and myoglobinuria who was found to have a partial deficiency of phosphofructokinase activity by biochemical assays.[70] Histochemical and ultrastructural studies on the muscle biopsy specimen from this patient revealed occasional degenerating and regenerating myofibers but no vacuoles, abnormal glycogen deposits, or polyglucosan bodies. In view of the varied clinical and morphologic manifestations of this disease, it is imperative that all patients who are even remotely suspected of phosphofructokinase deficiency be evaluated biochemically in a reference laboratory.

References

1. Biemond A, Daniels AP: Familial periodic paralysis and its transition into spinal muscular atrophy. Brain 57:91–108, 1934.
2. Tyler FH, Stephens FE, Gunn FD, Perkoff GT: Studies in disorders of muscle. VII. Clinical manifestations and inheritance of a type of periodic paralysis without hypopotassemia. J Clin Invest 30:492–502, 1951.
3. Gamstroph I: Adynamia episodica hereditaria. Acta Pediatr Scand 45 (Suppl 108):1–126, 1956.
4. Poskanzer DC, Kerr DNS: A third type of periodic paralysis, with normokalemia and favorable response to sodium chloride. Am J Med 31:328–342, 1961.
5. Brooke MH: A Clinician's View of Neuromuscular Diseases. Baltimore, Williams & Wilkins, 1977, p 188.
6. Meyers KR, Gilden DH, Rinaldi CF, Hansen JL: Periodic muscle weakness, normokalemia and tubular aggregates. Neurology 22: 269–279, 1972.
7. Chesson AL, Schochet SS Jr, Peters BH: Biphasic periodic paralysis. Arch Neurol 36:700–704, 1979.
8. Engel AG: Metabolic and endocrine myopathies. In Walton JN (ed): Disorders of Voluntary Muscle, 4th ed. Edinburgh, Churchill Livingstone, 1981, pp 664–711.
9. Pearson CM: The periodic paralyses: Differential features and pathological observations in permanent myopathic weakness. Brain 87:341–353, 1964.
10. Engel AG: Evolution and content of vacuoles in primary hypokalemic periodic paralysis. Mayo Clin Proc 45:774–814, 1970.
11. Schotland DL: An electron microscopic study of target fibers, target-like fibers and related abnormalities in human muscle. J Neuropathol Exp Neurol 28:214–228, 1969.
12. Schutta HS, Armitage JL: Thyrotoxic hypokalemic periodic paralysis: A fine structure study. J Neuropathol Exp Neurol 28: 321–326, 1969.

13. Takagi A, Schotland DL, DiMauro S, Rowland LP: Thyrotoxic periodic paralysis: Function of sarcoplasmic reticulum and muscle glycogen. Neurology 23:1008–1016, 1973.

14. Atsumi T, Ishikawa S, Miyatake T, Yoshida M: Myopathy and primary aldosteronism: Electronmicroscopic study. Neurology 29:1348–1353, 1979.

15. Engel WK, Bishop DW, Cunningham GG: Tubular aggregates in type II muscle fibers: Ultrastructural and histochemical correlation. J Ultrastruct Res 31:507–525, 1970.

16. Chui LA, Neustein H, Munsat TL: Tubular aggregates in subclinical alcoholic myopathy. Neurology 25:405–412, 1975.

17. Schroder JM, Becker PE: Anomalien des T-Systems und des sarkoplasmatischen Reticulums bei der Myotonie, Paramyotonie und Adynamie. Virchows Arch [A] 357:319–344, 1972.

18. Morgan-Hughes JA, Mair WGP, Lascelles PT: A disorder of skeletal muscle associated with tubular aggregates. Brain 93:873–880, 1970.

19. Lazaro RP, Fenichel GM, Kilroy AW, et al.: Cramps, muscle pain, and tubular aggregates. Arch Neurol 37:715–717, 1980.

20. Rohkamm R, Boxler K, Ricker K, Jerusalem F: A dominantly inherited myopathy with excessive tubular aggregates. Neurology 33:331–336, 1983.

21. Pierobon-Bormioli S, Armani M, Ringel SP, et al.: Familial neuromuscular disease with tubular aggregates. Muscle Nerve 8:291–298, 1985.

22. DiMauro S, Rowland LP, DiMauro PM: Control of glycogen metabolism in human muscle. Arch Neurol 23:534–540, 1970.

23. Essen B, Jansson E, Henriksson J, et al.: Metabolic characteristics of fibre types in human muscle. Acta Physiol Scand 95:153–165, 1975.

24. Vye MV, Fischman DA: The morphological alteration of particulate glycogen by *en bloc* staining with uranyl acetate. J Ultrast Res 33:278–291, 1970.

25. DiMauro S: Metabolic myopathies. In Vinken PJ, Bruyn GW (eds): Handbook of Clinical Neurology. Amsterdam, North-Holland, 1979, Vol 41, pp 175–234.

26. Wolfe HJ, Cohen RB: Nonglycogen polysaccharide storage in glycogenosis type II. Arch Pathol 86:579–584, 1968.

27. Schnabel R: Zur Histochemie der mucopolysaccharidartigen Substanzen (Basophilie Substanzen) in der Skeletmuskultur bei neuromuskularer Glykogenose (Typ II). Acta Neuropathol 17:169–178, 1971.

28. Sarnat HB, Roth SI, Carroll JE, et al.: Lipid storage myopathy in infantile Pompe's disease. Arch Neurol 39:180–183, 1982.

29. Engel AG, Gomez MR, Seybold ME, Lambert EH: The spectrum and diagnosis of acid maltase deficiency. Neurology 23:95–106, 1973.

30. Engel AG: Acid maltase deficiency in adults: Studies in four cases of a syndrome which may mimic muscular dystrophy or other myopathies. Brain 93:599–616, 1970.

31. McComas CF, Schochet SS Jr, Morris HH III, et al.: The constellation of adult acid maltase deficiency: Clinical, electrophysiologic, and morphologic features. J Clin Neuropathol 2:182–187, 1983.

32. Sivak ED, Salanga VD, Wilbourn AJ, et al.: Adult-onset acid maltase deficiency presenting as diaphragmatic paralysis. Ann Neurol 9:613–615, 1981.

33. Martin JJ, de Barsy T, den Tandt WR: Acid maltase deficiency in non-identical adult twins: Morphological and biochemical study. J Neurol 213:105–118, 1976.

34. Horoupian DS, Kini KR, Weiss L, Follmer R: Selective vacuolar myopathy with atrophy of type II fibers: Occurrence in a childhood case of acid maltase deficiency. Arch Neurol 35:175–178, 1978.

35. Karpati G, Carpenter S, Eisen A, et al.: The adult form of acid maltase (α-1,4-glucosidase) deficiency. Ann Neurol 1:276–280, 1977.
36. Martin JJ, de Barsy T, de Schrijver F, et al.: Acid maltase deficiency (type II glycogenosis). Morphological and biochemical study of a childhood phenotype. J Neurol Sci 30:155–166, 1976.
37. Engel AG, Dale AJD: Autophagic glycogenosis of late onset with mitochondrial abnormalities: Light and electron microscopic observations. Mayo Clin Proc 43:233–279, 1968.
38. Dreyfus JC: Glycogen storage diseases. Pathobiol Annu 4:289–313, 1974.
39. Angelini C, Engel AG: Comparative study of acid maltase deficiency. Arch Neurol 26:344–349, 1972.
40. Miranda AF, Shanske S, Hays AP, DiMauro S: Immunocytochemical analysis of normal and acid maltase deficient muscle cultures. Arch Neurol 42:371–373, 1985.
41. DiMauro S, Stern LZ, Mehler M, et al.: Adult-onset acid maltase deficiency. A postmortem study. Muscle Nerve 1:27–36, 1978.
42. Loonen MCB, Busch HFM, Koster JF, et al.: A family with different clinical forms of acid maltase deficiency (glycogenosis type II): Biochemical and genetic studies. Neurology 31:1209–1216, 1981.
43. Danon MJ, Oh SJ, DiMauro S, et al.: Lysosomal glycogen storage disease with normal acid maltase. Neurology 31:51–57, 1981.
44. Riggs JE, Schochet SS Jr, Gutmann L, et al.: Lysosomal glycogen storage disease without acid maltase deficiency. Neurology 33:873–877, 1983.
45. Brown BI, Brown DH: Glycogen-storage diseases: Types I, III, IV, V, VII and unclassified glycogenoses. In Dicken F, Randle PJ, Whelan W (eds): Carbohydrate Metabolism and Its Disorders. New York, Academic Press, 1968, Vol 2, pp 123–150.
46. Pellissier JF, de Barsy T, Faugere MC, Rebuffel P: Type III glycogenosis with multicore structures. Muscle Nerve 2:124–132, 1979.
47. Brunberg JA, McCormick WF, Schochet SS Jr: Type III glycogenosis: An adult with diffuse weakness and muscle wasting. Arch Neurol 25:171–178, 1971.
48. DiMauro S, Hartwig GB, Hays A, et al.: Debrancher deficiency. Neuromuscular disorder in 5 adults. Ann Neurol 5:422–436, 1979.
49. Cornelio F, Bresolin N, Singer PA, et al.: Clinical varieties of neuromuscular disease in debrancher deficiency. Arch Neurol 41:1027–1032, 1984.
50. Mercier C, Whelan WJ: The fine structure of glycogen from type IV glycogen-storage disease. Eur J Biochem 16:579–583, 1970.
51. Zellweger H, Mueller S, Ionasescu V, et al.: Glycogenosis IV: A new cause of infantile hypotonia. J Pediatr 80:842–844, 1972.
52. Schochet SS Jr, McCormick WF, Zellweger H: Type IV glycogenosis (amylopectinosis). Arch Pathol 90:354–363, 1970.
53. Bannayan GA, Dean WJ, Howell RR: Type IV glcogen-storage disease: Light-microscopic, electron-microscopic and enzymatic study. Am J Clin Pathol 66:702–709, 1976.
54. McMaster KR, Powers JM, Hennigar GR Jr, et al.: Nervous system involvement in type IV glycogenosis. Arch Pathol Lab Med 103:105–111, 1970.
55. Schochet SS Jr, McCormick WF, Kovarsky J: Light and electron microscopy of skeletal muscle in type IV glycogenosis. Acta Neuropathol 19:137–144, 1971.
56. Feit H, Brooke MH: Myophosphorylase deficiency: Two different molecular etiologies. Neurology 26:963–967, 1976.
57. Kost GJ, Verity MA: A new variant of late-onset myophosphorylase deficiency. Muscle Nerve 3:195–201, 1980.

58. Engel WK, Eyerman EL, Williams HE: Late-onset type of skeletal-muscle phosphorylase deficiency. N Engl J Med 268:135–137, 1963.

59. DiMauro S, Hartlage PL: Fatal infantile form of muscle phosphorylase deficiency. Neurology 28:1124–1129, 1978.

60. Miranda AF, Nette EG, Hartlage PL, DiMauro S: Phosphorylase isoenzymes in normal and myophosphorylase-deficient human heart. Neurology 29:1538–1541, 1979.

61. Cornelio F, Bresolin N, DiMauro S, et al.: Congenital myopathy due to phosphorylase deficiency. Neurology 33:1383–1385, 1983.

62. Schotland DL, Spiro D, Rowland LP, Carmel P: Ultrastructural studies of muscle in McArdle's disease. J Neuropathol Exp Neurol 24:629–644, 1965.

63. Layzer RB, Rowland LP, Ranney HM: Muscle phosphofructokinase deficiency. Arch Neurol 17:512–523, 1967.

64. Mineo I, Kono N, Schimizu T, et al.: A comparative study on glucagon effect between McArdle disease and Tarui disease. Muscle Nerve 7:552–559, 1984.

65. Penn AS: Myoglobin and myoglobinuria. In Viken PJ, Bruyn GW (eds): Handbook of Clinical Neurology. Amsterdam, North-Holland, 1979, Vol 41, pp 259–285.

66. Hays AP, Hallet M, Delfs J, et al.: Muscle phosphofructokinase deficiency: Abnormal polysaccharide in a case of late-onset myopathy. Neurology 31:1077–1086, 1981.

67. Danon MJ, Carpenter S, Manaligod JR, Schlisefeld LH: Fatal infantile glycogen storage disease: Deficiency of phosphofructokinase and phosphorylase b kinase. Neurology 31:1303–1307, 1981.

68. Bonilla E, Schotland DL: Histochemical diagnosis of muscle phosphofructokinase deficiency. Arch Neurol 22:8–12, 1970.

69. Agamanolis DP, Askari AD, DiMauro S, et al.: Muscle phosphofructokinase deficiency: Two cases with unusual polysaccharide accumulation and immunologically active enzyme protein. Muscle Nerve 3:456–467, 1980.

70. DiMauro S: Personal communication.

chapter 7

Lipid Myopathies, Mitochondrial Myopathies, and Other Metabolic Myopathies

As indicated in Chapter 6, lipids are important substrates for metabolism by skeletal muscle at rest and during sustained exercise.[1] Prior to oxidation within mitochondria, lipids must undergo a series of preliminary reactions in order to pass through the mitochondrial membranes. Carnitine serves as an obligatory carrier for the passage of long-chain fatty acid residues through the inner mitochondrial membrane. The carnitine used in these reactions is synthesized predominantly in the liver and actively transported into the muscle. Intracellular free fatty acids, derived from circulating lipids and endogenous triglycerides are converted to acyl-coenzyme A (acyl-CoA) compounds by the action of fatty acyl-CoA synthetase. The acyl-CoA compounds are bound to carnitine by various acylcarnitine transferases such as carnitine pamityltransferase. This reaction occurs predominantly on the outer surface of the inner mitochondrial membrane. After passage through the mitochondrial membrane, other acylcarnitine transferases, located on the inner surface of the inner mitochondrial membrane, free the acyl-CoA compounds from the carnitine. Only after these steps are the lipids able to undergo beta oxidation within the mitochondrial matrix space and provide energy for use by the muscle.

LIPID IN NORMAL SKELETAL MUSCLE

Some of the fatty acids utilized by skeletal muscle are derived from triglycerides stored in the form of intracellular lipid droplets. These are usually evaluated morphologically in frozen sections stained by oil red O (Fig. 7–1). The staining

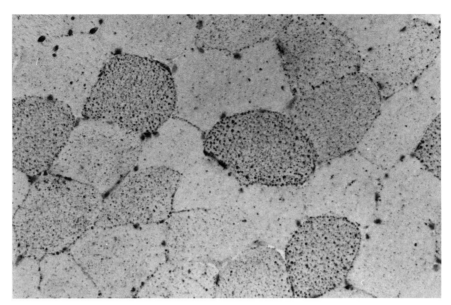

Figure 7-1. Frozen section stained with oil red O. The type I myofibers normally contain more numerous and larger lipid droplets than the type II myofibers. ×430.

depends on selective extraction of the dye by the lipid droplets from the stain solution. Often these preparations are difficult to interpret because of extraneous dye deposits on the surface of the sections. We have found that staining with osmium tetroxide, followed by paraphenylenediamine (Fig. 7-2) often yields cleaner results although the staining is not confined to triglyceride droplets. Regardless of the technique, lipid droplets appear larger and more numerous in type I myofibers but are not especially conspicuous in normal muscle. By electron microscopy, the triglyceride deposits appear as unstained or weakly osmiophilic rounded droplets. They have smooth margins and are not membrane bounded. The lipid droplets are most numerous beneath the sarcolemma adjacent to the myofiber nuclei and in rows between the myofibrils. The droplets are often immediately adjacent to mitochondria. Biochemical studies on individual myofibers have shown that type I myofibers normally contain about three times more triglyceride than type II myofibers.[2]

LIPID MYOPATHIES

General

The histologic demonstration of excessive numbers of lipid droplets in muscle biopsy specimens provided the initial evidence that human muscle diseases could result from abnormal lipid metabolism.[3,4] The patients described in the

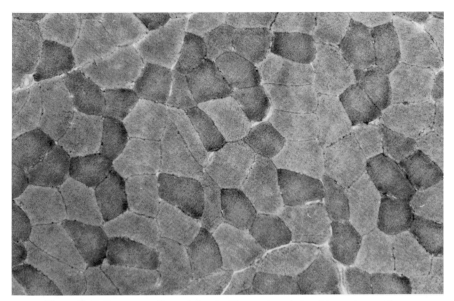

Figure 7-2. Frozen section stained with osmium tetroxide and paraphenylenediamine. The preparations are cleaner but the staining is less specific for triglycerides. × 170.

earlier reports displayed disparate clinical manifestations. Some had progressive proximal muscle weakness[3] while others had recurrent cramps and myoglobinuria.[4] Biochemical studies on subsequent patients firmly established disorders of lipid metabolism as a distinct category of muscle disease. At the present time, the more clearly delineated lipid myopathies result from deficient interactions between carnitine and free fatty acid residues.[1] The diseases include two forms of primary carnitine deficiency, myopathic and systemic, and deficiency of carnitine palmityltransferase activity. Myopathies also may result from secondary carnitine deficiency and other defective steps in lipid metabolism.

Primary Carnitine Deficiencies

Two more or less distinct disorders have been associated with a primary deficiency of carnitine. So-called "myopathic" carnitine deficiency was delineated biochemically in 1973 by Engel and Angelini.[5] In this condition, muscle carnitine levels are markedly reduced while the liver, and plasma carnitine levels are normal or only slightly decreased. The intramuscular carnitine deficiency has been attributed to impaired active transport of this compound into the muscle. The disease begins in childhood or early adult life and is characterized by progressive proximal muscle weakness.

Muscle biopsy specimens from these patients display an increased number of lipid droplets especially in type I myofibers. Ultrastructural studies have shown that the abnormal lipid accumulation is accompanied by minimal or no increase in the number of mitochondria. In some cases, however, the mitochondria have shown mild structural alterations such as indistinct cristae, abnormally arranged cristae, and intracristal paracrystalline arrays.[6,7] In at least one case, lipid droplets were also encountered in Schwann cells and in leukocytes.[8]

So-called "systemic" carnitine deficiency was first reported by Karpati et al. in 1975.[9] In this condition, plasma, hepatic and muscle carnitine levels are reduced. This disease becomes manifest in infancy or childhood and is more severe than myopathic carnitine deficiency. In systemic carnitine deficiency, proximal muscle weakness is accompanied or preceded by episodes of hepatic and cerebral dysfunction that may resemble Reye's syndrome.[10] Myocardial involvement may lead to death during childhood or early adult life. Endocardial fibroelastosis has been described in three children from a family with this disorder.[11]

Muscle biopsy specimens from patients with systemic carnitine deficiency show a prominent increase in the number of lipid droplets. These are found mainly within type I myofibers. However, the type I myofibers are not uniformly affected. Preferential involvement of a specific subtype of the type I myofibers has been suggested.[12] Ultrastructural studies have shown a mild increase in the number of mitochondria along with excessively numerous lipid droplets. Generally, the mitochondria show only minimal structural abnormalities. However, abundant giant mitochondria, intramitochondrial dense bodies, and intracristal paracrystalline arrays were encountered in the patients reported by Boudin et al.[13] and Engel et al.[14] The systemic nature of this disease is reflected morphologically by increased lipid in myocardium, liver, and kidneys. The disease had been attributed to deficient hepatic synthesis of carnitine. More recent studies[15,16] have challenged this view and have suggested that there is impaired carnitine uptake by multiple organs along with excessive renal excretion of this compound.

Still other cases of lipid storage myopathy have mixed features of both the "myopathic" and the "systemic" forms of primary carnitine deficiency.[12,17] Some of these individuals have low serum carnitine levels but no evidence of liver disease while others have normal serum carnitine levels and clinical manifestations that are more consistent with the systemic form of the disease.

Secondary Carnitine Deficiency

Reduced serum and/or muscle carnitine levels have been encountered in association with other diseases. These have included schistosomiasis, sepsis, and certain mitochondrial myopathies. Reduced carnitine levels are also found in patients on hemodialysis for renal failure.[17] Muscle specimens from some of these patients have shown abnormal lipid accumulations. We studied a woman with neuropathy and myopathy following a gastric plication for morbid obesity.[18] She had a mildly reduced serum carnitine level and a mild increase in the number of lipid droplets in type I myofibers (Fig. 7–3).

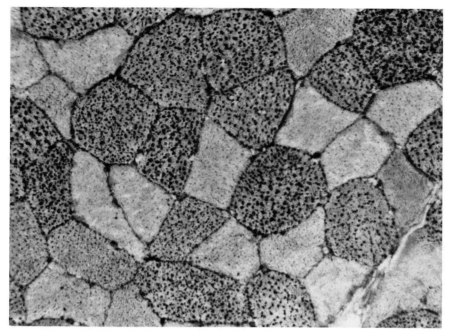

Figure 7-3. Muscle biopsy specimen from a 27-year-old woman who was found to have mildly reduced serum carnitine levels, myopathy, and neuropathy subsequent to a gastric plication. Note the increased numbers of lipid droplets in the type I myofibers. Paraphenylenediamine, ×440.

Carnitine Palmityltransferase Deficiency

Carnitine palmityltransferase deficiency was originally described in 1973 by DiMauro and DiMauro.[19] Males are affected far more often than females. Patients with this disorder often have recurrent episodes of rhabdomyolysis and myoglobinuria dating back to childhood. Most of the episodes of rhabdomyolysis are precipitated by strenuous exercise, especially when combined with exposure to cold or after fasting. The patients have no difficulty with mild exercise and do not develop cramps or contractures. In contrast to some of the glycogenoses, lactate is produced normally during ischemic exercise testing. Some of the patients have strikingly elevated plasma triglyceride levels and decreased ketone production during prolonged fasting.

Muscle biopsy specimens from asymptomatic patients with carnitine palmityltransferase deficiency generally show no abnormalities. Scattered necrotic myofibers and an increased number of lipid droplets may be encountered if the biopsy is obtained during an episode of rhabdomyolysis. Lipid storage is far less conspicuous than in the carnitine deficiency states. Increased numbers of lipid droplets have been observed in less than one third of the reported cases of carnitine palmityltransferase deficiency.[17] The explanation for this striking contrast is unknown.

Other Lipid Myopathies

There are other, less well delineated lipid myopathies, that are apparently not due to abnormalities in carnitine metabolism. One such disease is the lipid storage myopathy associated with congenital ichthyosis.[20,21] Muscle biopsy specimens from these patients have disclosed increased numbers of lipid droplets in type I myofibers. Excess lipid is also present in numerous other tissues including liver, intestinal mucosa, fibroblasts, and leukocytes. There is no associated glycogen storage and no mitochondrial abnormalities are evident by electron microscopy. A defect in triglyceride utilization has been suggested but the metabolic basis for this entity has not been fully elucidated. Another example of lipid storage myopathy unrelated to carnitine metabolism was reported by Jerusalem et al.[22] Their patient was a 28-year-old woman with nonprogressive muscular weakness who had been hypotonic as an infant. Muscle biopsy specimens disclosed large numbers of lipid droplets in both type I and type II myofibers. Electron microscopy showed approximately a hundredfold increase in lipid but no significant abnormalities in the morphology of the mitochondria. Both serum and muscle carnitine levels and muscle carnitine palmityltransferase activity were normal. Under the name of mitochondria-lipid–glycogen disease, Jerusalem et al.[23] described a 7-month-old infant with hypotonia, hyporeflexia, hepatomegaly, and macroglossia. Muscle biopsy specimens revealed numerous lipid droplets, abundant glycogen granules, and myriads of mildly dysmorphic mitochondria. Despite the severity of the initial manifestations, the child improved clinically and the morphologic abnormalities had regressed by the age of 22 months. The muscle carnitine level and oxidation of oleate were normal. Askanas et al.[24] recently have described a lipid neuromyopathy in a woman and her two sons. Biopsy specimens showed mild type II myofiber atrophy and increased lipid in type I myofibers and Schwann cells. Carnitine levels and carnitine palmityltransferase activities were normal. The patients showed clinical improvement and resolution of morphologic abnormalities with a long-chain fatty-acid-free diet.

Occasionally lipid storage may be encountered in muscle specimens from patients with other categories of metabolic disease. Sarnat et al.[25] recently reported abundant lipid storage in an infant with otherwise typical Pompe's disease. Less conspicuous accumulation of lipid also has been described in adult-onset acid maltase disease.[26]

MITOCHONDRIAL MYOPATHIES

The diagnostic limitations of morphology are probably more evident among the so-called "mitochondrial myopathies" than in any other group of neuromuscular diseases. The concept of abnormal mitochondrial function as the basis for muscular disease was introduced by Luft et al.[27] These workers described a young woman with heat intolerance, polydipsia, hyperphagia, and increased basal metabolic rate. The authors demonstrated that this hypermetabolic state resulted from a defect of respiratory control in skeletal muscle mitochondria rather than from thyroid dysfunction. In the original case and a subsequent case[28,29] of "Luft's disease," the biochemical abnormalities were accompanied by morphologic abnormalities consisting of excessively numerous large mitochondria with aberrant cristae. Subsequently, abnormal mitochondrial number, size, and shape were the major criteria for delineation of disorders such as megaconial myopathy[30] and pleoconial myopathy.[31] These terms are no longer used since it is now recognized that morphologic features alone are inadequate criteria for identifying or distinguishing mitochondrial myopathies.[32] Some diseases that clearly result from disorders of mitochondrial metabolism, such as the carnitine myopathies, show few or no morphologic abnormalities among the mitochondria. Conversely, at least mild mitochondrial structural abnormalities have been seen in association with a wide variety of muscular diseases in which significant errors of mitochondrial metabolism have not yet been implicated. These include denervation, inflammatory myopathies, dystrophies, and diverse metabolic disorders.

Despite these diagnostic limitations, it is important to recognize and properly evaluate the morphologic manifestations of mitochondrial abnormalities. In some instances, they indicate the need for more extensive biochemical evaluation in order to establish a definitive diagnosis. In a few cases, the morphologic findings in conjunction with the clinical data can provide a reasonably certain diagnosis. In still other instances, the mitochondrial abnormalities must be regarded as coincidental findings of undetermined significance. These judgments are based on the extent of the mitochondrial alterations and the presence or absence of other associated morphologic aberrations.

By light microscopy, mitochondrial abnormalities are far more readily evaluated in frozen sections than in paraffin-embedded sections. Myofibers with abnormal accumulations of mitochondria display subsarcolemmal and intermyofibrillar deposits of granular material that stain blue with H&E and red with the modified trichrome stain (Fig. 7–4). The fibers harboring the abnormal deposits of mitochondria are generally called "ragged-red" fibers, a term that was introduced by Olson et al.[33] The fibers so affected are most often type I myofibers. They may also contain increased numbers of lipid droplets. Since accumulations of materials other than mitochondria may simulate "ragged-red" fibers, the identification of deposits suspected of being mitochondria should be confirmed histochemically by the use of oxidative enzyme stains. The succinic dehydrogenase stain is commonly employed for this purpose. With this procedure, mitochondrial deposits stain darkly. Mitochondrial deposits also stain darkly with the NADH–TR reaction. This reaction, however, is less specific since normal and abnormal components of the sarcoplasmic reticulum also stain darkly with this technique.

A wide variety of mitochondrial abnormalities may be seen by electron microscopy. Mitochondria with apparently normal ultrastructure simply may be present in excessive numbers. Other mitochondria may be abnormally large or may display aberrant orientation of their cristae (Figs. 7–5 and 7–6). By far,

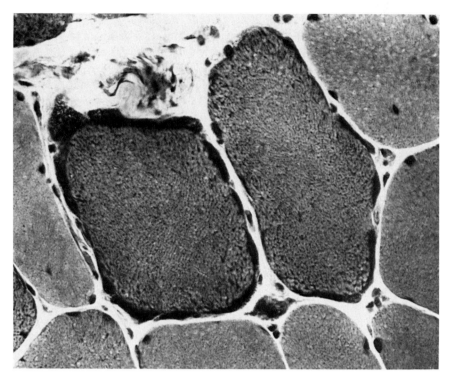

Figure 7-4. Muscle biopsy specimen from a 40-year-old woman with ocu-lopharyngeal dystrophy. Abnormal deposits of mitochondria appear as discontinuous irregular red bands at the periphery of type I myofibers. Trichrome, ×600.

the most spectacular of the mitochondrial structural abnormalities is the presence of rectangular paracrystalline inclusions (Fig. 7–7). These are located within the intracristal spaces and between the inner and outer mitochondrial membranes. The paracrystalline masses are composed of sets of parallel osmiophilic lines with periodic punctate densities (Fig. 7–8). In transverse section, each set appears to be formed by four parallel lines. The osmiophilic densities are alternately situated between the first and second lines and between the third and fourth lines. These inclusions are sometimes described as resembling a "parking lot." Relatively little is known about the chemical composition and pathogenesis of these paracrystalline structures. It has even been suggested that they may be biochemically inert.[34] Somewhat similar inclusions have been produced experimentally by the in vivo infusion of uncoupling agents or oleic acid.[35]

Conditions with Morphologic Mitochondrial Abnormalities
As mentioned previously, there is limited correlation between morphologically demonstrated mitochondrial abnormalities and biochemically delineated abnormalities of mitochondrial metabolism, i.e., the true mitochondrial myopa-

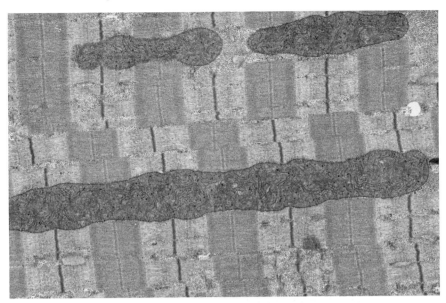

Figure 7-5. Muscle biopsy specimen from an 11-year-old mentally retarded boy with proximal muscle weakness. Note the abnormally large mitochondria extended over multiple sarcomeres. ×13,125.

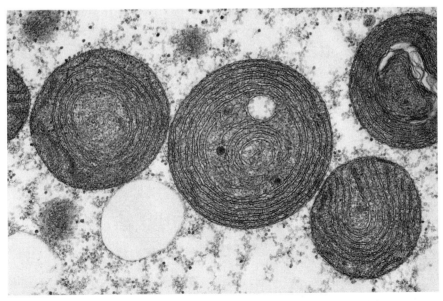

Figure 7-6. Muscle biopsy specimen from a 40-year-old woman with oculopharyngeal dystrophy. Note the aberrant orientation of the mitochondrial cristae. ×58,000.

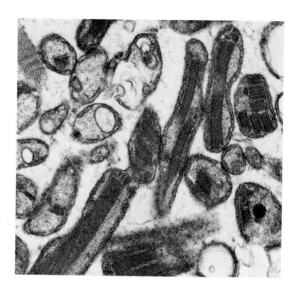

Figure 7-7. Muscle biopsy specimen from an 18-year-old woman with the Kearns–Sayre syndrome. Note the rectangular paracrystalline inclusions in many of the abnormal mitochondria. ×28,000.

thies. Nevertheless, it is important for the morphologist to be familiar with the spectrum of conditions in which mitochondrial structural abnormalities may be seen by light or electron microscopy. The reader is referred to chapters by DiMauro[1] and Morgan-Hughes[32] for further discussion from a biochemical point of view.

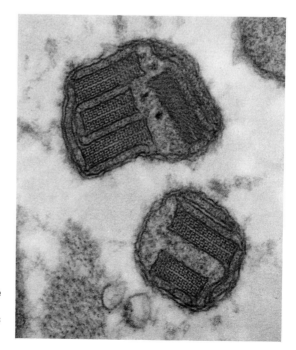

Figure 7-8. The inclusions are composed of a set of parallel osmiophilic lines and periodic punctate densities. ×72,000.

Hypermetabolic States Including Luft's Disease. Although this is the paradigm of the true mitochondrial myopathies, only two patients with the fully expressed disease have been reported to date.[27-29] Both were women with heat intolerance, excessive sweating, dyspnea, polyphagia, and polydipsia. Both had markedly increased basal metabolic rates but normal thyroid function. They showed only mild to moderate muscular weakness. Muscle biopsy specimens showed excessively numerous mitochondria with mild structural abnormalities. No other significant morphologic abnormalities were evident in the muscle. Biochemical studies demonstrated loose coupling, i.e., impaired control of mitochondrial respiration by phosphorylation.[27] Further biochemical studies on the second patient suggested that abnormalities in the mitochondrial retention of calcium may have been responsible for the loose coupling.[29] Carpenter and Karpati have indicated that there are additional patients with incomplete manifestations of this syndrome.[36]

Abnormalities of Pyruvate Metabolism. A wide spectrum of neurologic disorders have been attributed to abnormalities in the metabolism of pyruvate.[37] These have included microcephaly, psychomotor retardation, hypotonia, lactic acidosis, Leigh's syndrome in infancy, and various forms of hereditary ataxia in older children and adults. Some of these associations have been disputed by other workers. Muscle biopsy specimens from a few patients with cerebellar ataxia and some patients with Leigh's disease[38] have shown mitochondrial abnormalities including "ragged-red" fibers.

Disorders of Lipid Metabolism. Although the lipid myopathies meet biochemical criteria for true mitochondrial myopathies, morphologic abnormalities among the mitochondria generally are relatively inconspicuous. As previously mentioned, mitochondrial abnormalities are usually more conspicuous in specimens from patients with myopathic carnitine deficiency than in specimens from patients with systemic carnitine deficiency.

Disorders of Mitochondrial Respiratory Chain Enzymes. A heterogenous group of neurologic disorders has been associated with abnormalities in mitochondrial oxidative metabolism. Most often, these have involved dysfunction of the portions of the respiratory chain measured by NADH–cytochrome-c-reductase or cytochrome-c-oxidase.[1,32] In a few cases the metabolic defect has involved succinate–cytochrome-c-reductase activity.[39]

Several of these patients included in this heterogeneous group have presented in infancy with varying combinations of psychomotor retardation, weakness, lethargy, metabolic acidosis, and respiratory distress.[40] Some of the older children have displayed neurosensory hearing loss and optic atrophy but normal intellectual function. Among the adults, weakness, exercise intolerance, ataxia, and even dementia have been reported. Not all of the patients have had clinical myopathy. Muscle specimens have shown varying numbers of "ragged-red" myofibers by light microscopy (Figs. 7–9 and 7–10) and increased num-

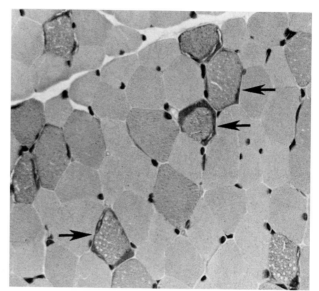

Figure 7-9. Muscle biopsy specimen from a 9-year-old girl with a mitochondrial encephalomyopathy with decreased succinate-cytochrome-c-reductase.[39] Abnormal deposits of mitochondria appear as basophilic bands at the periphery of type I myofibers *(arrows).* H&E, ×410.

bers of mitochondria with diverse structural anomalies by electron microscopy. Some have also shown increased glycogen and/or lipid deposits (Fig. 7–11). All of these diseases are rare and many have been reported as unique entities.

Mitochondrial Myopathy in Association with External Ophthalmoplegia. This category includes cases of the Kearns–Sayre syndrome and familial ophthalmoplegic syndromes. The Kearns–Sayre syndrome is generally regarded as a

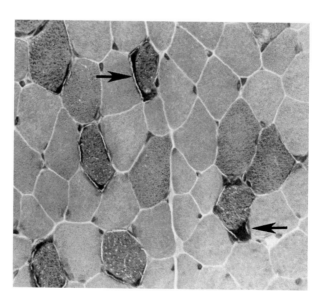

Figure 7-10. Same patient as in Figure 7-9. The abnormal deposits of mitochondria *(arrows)* are stained bright red by the modified trichrome procedure. ×410.

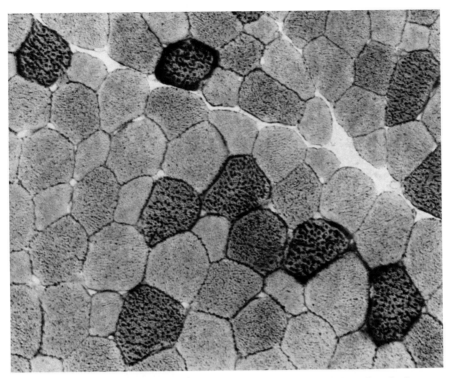

Figure 7-11. Same patient as in Figure 7-9. The abnormal deposits of mitochondria are accompanied by an increased number of large lipid droplets in type I myofibers. Note that both the lipid droplets and mitochondrial deposits are stained. Os–PPD, ×410.

sporadic multisystem disorder. Ophthalmoplegia, pigmentary degeneration of the retina, heart block, and increased cerebrospinal fluid protein are among the most consistent features.[1,41,42] The disease has its onset in childhood or adolescence and usually is apparent before the age of 20. Other clinical features that occasionally may be present include short stature, cerebellar ataxia, impaired hearing, vestibular dysfunction, intellectual impairment, and peripheral neuropathy. Death often results from the cardiac conduction defects.[43]

Muscle specimens from patients with the Kearns–Sayre syndrome have shown few to many "ragged-red" myofibers. Diverse ultrastructural abnormalities, including numerous intracristal paracrystalline arrays, are encountered among the mitochondria (see Figs. 7–7 and 7–8). Similar mitochondrial abnormalities have been demonstrated in other tissues including liver,[44] skin,[41] and brain.[45] Biochemical studies have failed to demonstrate a consistent metabolic derangement. Some authors have even suggested that these mitochondrial abnormalities are acquired, possibly as the result of a chronic viral infection.

Muscle specimens from patients with oculopharyngeal dystrophy and other familial ocular myopathies also display various mitochondrial abnormalities.[46] These cases are distinguished clinically by their later age of onset and lack of the systemic features that are usually encountered in the Kearns–Sayre syndrome.

Mitochondrial Abnormalities in Other Diseases. Emphasizing the nonspecificity of the mitochondrial abnormalities is the fact that occasional "ragged-red" myofibers and abnormal accumulations of mitochondria may be encountered in a wide variety of diseases, including cases of facioscapulohumeral dystrophy, myotonic dystrophy, inclusion body myositis, and neurogenic atrophy. We have even encountered abundant mitochondrial deposits in a child with hypomagnesemia (Fig. 7–12).

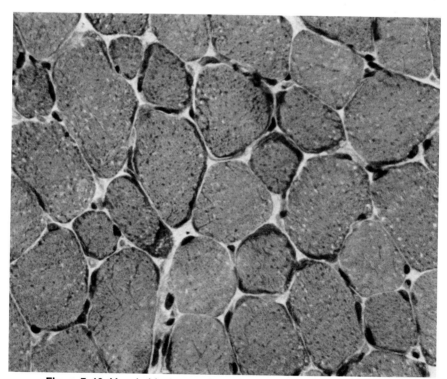

Figure 7-12. Muscle biopsy specimen from a boy with hypertrophic cardiomyopathy, proximal myopathy, and hypomagnesemia. Note the numerous myofibers that are encircled by abnormal basophilic deposits containing mitochondria. H&E, ×410.

ENDOCRINE MYOPATHIES

Despite the prominence of muscular weakness in association with many endocrinologic disorders, there are few well-documented morphologic alterations. Of these, mild myofiber atrophy is the most consistently encountered.

Proximal muscular weakness and wasting, affecting especially the lower limbs, may be seen in association with excess corticosteroids. This can be seen in Cushing's disease, and even more commonly in individuals receiving exogenous corticosteroids. The predominant histopathologic alteration in muscle specimens from these individuals is type II myofiber atrophy (see Fig. 2–20). Often the type IIB myofibers appear to be the more severely affected. The precise relations between dose and duration of drug administration in iatrogenic steroid myopathy have not been well established. Type II myofiber atrophy may be seen even in the absence of clinically manifest myopathy. Occasionally, an increased number of lipid droplets may be seen in the type I myofibers. This has been reported to be an earlier manifestation of the steroid excess.[47] Other degenerative changes have been reported but are uncommon and less well documented. By electron microscopy, there may be an apparent increase in glycogen content. Whether this is due to the steroid-induced increase in glycogen synthetase activity or is merely the result of atrophy, i.e., loss of contractile elements, is unsettled.

Although patients with hyperthyroidism often have generalized muscular weakness and may have elevated serum muscle enzymes, muscle specimens are usually normal or show only mild myofiber atrophy by light microscopy. Ultrastructurally, abnormal papillary projections containing mitochondria and glycogen have been reported on the surface of myofibers but are probably nonspecific manifestations of myofiber atrophy.[48] Occasional patients, especially Oriental males, may develop thyrotoxic periodic paralysis. As in other types of periodic paralysis, muscle specimens from these individuals may contain tubular aggregates. Mitochondrial abnormalities, including intracristal paracrystalline arrays and intracytoplasmic cylindrical filamentous bodies, also have been reported.[49]

Patients with hypothyroidism may have muscle stiffness and delayed relaxation of deep tendon reflexes. Some have hypertrophy of the calves and thighs. Muscle specimens usually show only mild type II myofiber atrophy and an increased glycogen content. Basophilic degeneration of skeletal muscle, comparable to basophilic degeneration of the myocardium by both light and electron microscopy, has been reported in association with long-standing hypothyroidism.[50,51]

Muscular weakness in at least some patients with hyperparathyroidism is due to a neurogenic disorder that resembles motor neuron disease.[52] Muscle specimens from these individuals showed type II myofiber atrophy and manifestations of denervation, i.e., small angular myofibers of both major fiber types and occasional target fibers.

MYONECROSIS AND RHABDOMYOLYSIS

There are a wide variety of circumstances in which skeletal muscle is damaged sufficiently for the myofibers to undergo necrosis. The process can involve whole muscles or scattered individual fibers. The term "rhabdomyolysis" is often employed to indicate widespread necrosis of individual myofibers rather than whole muscles. Generally, many of the affected myofibers appear to be at a similar stage of injury and may be degenerating or undergoing phagocytosis (Fig. 7–13). The phagocytes in the fibers undergoing myophagocytosis show prominent nonspecific esterase activity. In at least some patients, there appears to be preferential involvement of one fiber type, e.g., type I myofiber involvement in rhabdomyolysis associated with epsilon-aminocaproic acid (EACA) therapy.[53] If sufficient time has elapsed between the episode of rhabdomyolysis and histologic examination, many of the fibers will show evidence of concurrent regeneration. The regenerating fibers are amphophilic and contain large nuclei (Fig. 7–14). In most cases inflammation is remarkably sparse. If the rhabdomyolytic process is recurrent, one may encounter foci of mineralization as sequelae of prior episodes of remote necrosis.

One of the consequences of severe muscle fiber injury and necrosis is the release of myoglobin into the circulation. This relatively small molecule is readily cleared by the kidney and appears in the urine, i.e., myoglobinuria. The myoglobinuria may be severe enough to produce grossly discolored urine or

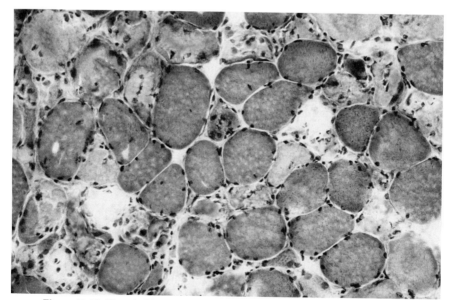

Figure 7–13. Muscle biopsy specimen from a 20-year-old woman who developed rhabdomyolysis while being treated with epsilon-aminocaproic acid. Note the widespread necrosis of myofibers. H&E, ×240.

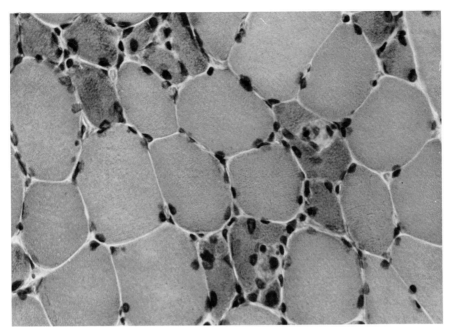

Figure 7-14. Muscle biopsy specimen from a patient recovering from rhabdomyolysis for which the etiology was undetermined. Note the numerous amphophilic myofibers with relative large vesicular nuclei characteristic of regeneration. H&E, ×440.

may be detectable only by chemical, spectroscopic, or immunologic analysis. In some circumstances the myoglobinuria may be sufficient to lead to renal failure.

Among the many recognized causes of myoglobinuria are direct musculoskeletal trauma, ischemia, overexertion, intoxications, inflammatory disorders, and metabolic derangements.[54] In addition, there remains an idiopathic category for which the cause cannot be elucidated. Massive necrosis of skeletal muscles with associated myoglobinuria may result from traumatic crushing injuries or the indirect crushing of dependent portions of the body in a comatose patient. Under these circumstances, the necrosis is due, at least in part, to impaired circulation with prolonged ischemia of muscle. Conversely, myonecrosis has been observed in various forms of extreme exertion. This has been observed in military recruits who have engaged in strenuous exercise, especially in hot weather.[55] The "anterior tibial syndrome," observed following prolonged marches, is often included among the exercise-induced forms of myoglobinuria but is probably due, at least in part, to localized muscle ischemia.[56] A somewhat similar pattern of myonecrosis, confined to abdominal wall muscles, has been reported in association with "body building" exercises.[57] Seizures are another cause of exertional rhabdomyolysis. They were considered to be the third most common cause of rhabdomyolysis in a series of 77 civilian cases studied by Gabow et al.[58]

Rhabdomyolysis has been attributed to many different toxins, ranging from exotic entities such as sea snake venom to common substances such as alcohol. Alcohol was regarded as the most common etiologic factor in the series of 77 cases published by Gabow et al.[58] Although these authors' criteria for implicating alcohol were quite liberal, alcohol is clearly an important cause of rhabdomyolysis. Acute alcoholic myopathy usually develops abruptly following a period of heavy alcohol consumption. The patients have proximal muscle weakness and tenderness that affects the upper limbs more than the lower limbs. In other individuals, alcohol may produce a painless myopathy accompanied by hypokalemia.[59] In these patients, there is vacuolar degeneration in addition to the scattered necrotic myofibers. In view of the association between hypokalemia and at least some forms of alcoholic myopathy, it is of interest to note that tubular aggregates have been described in a subclinical case of alcoholic myopathy.[60]

A wide variety of drugs, including both common therapeutic agents and abused substances, are known to produce toxic myopathies that may be accompanied by rhabdomyolysis.[54,58] Among these are amphetamines, amphotericin, barbiturates, EACA, heroin, methadone, phencyclidine, and succinylcholine.

Among the metabolic diseases, myophosphorylase deficiency, phosphofructokinase deficiency, and carnitine palmityltransferase deficiency are the ones most often responsible for rhabdomyolysis. DiMauro[1] has suggested that carnitine palmityltransferase deficiency may be the most common cause of hereditary rhabdomyolysis. These metabolic diseases share in common inadequate substrate utilization for energy production.

Several viral infections have been implicated in causing rhabdomyolysis. In some cases, the evidence is based on the concurrent association with rising antibody titers. In a few patients, virus particles have been visualized by electron microscopy or isolated from muscle. Gamboa et al.[61] reported rhabdomyolysis in a patient with a subacute myopathy. Although the case had many features of dermatomyositis, influenza B virus was isolated from the muscle. In such cases, the possibility of coexistent metabolic diseases or toxic exposure also must be considered.

MISCELLANEOUS TOXIC MYOPATHIES

A wide variety of compounds, including certain drugs, may produce toxic myopathies with a milder degree of myofiber damage rather than rhabdomyolysis. Chloroquine, a quinoline used as an antimalarial and in the treatment of certain collagen–vascular diseases such as lupus, is such a compound. The chronic administration of this drug is known to produce widespread, slowly progressive weakness.[62] Histologic studies on patients with this condition have shown a vacuolar myopathy in which the vacuoles may be partially filled with PAS-positive material.[63] These are found predominantly in type I myofibers. An experimental study by MacDonald and Engel[64] showed that the vacuoles resulted from focal autophagic degradation of the muscle fibers. The membranes comprising the autophagic vacuoles were derived from proliferation of the sarcoplasmic reticulum and T-tubules. Residual bodies, containing curvilinear profiles that closely resemble the inclusions seen in neuronal ceroid lipofuscinosis, may persist in the muscle for years following chloroquine therapy.[65] This must be considered when muscle biopsy specimens are being evaluated to establish a morphologic diagnosis of Kufs' disease, the adult form of neuronal ceroid lipofuscinosis.

Colchicine, used in the therapy of gout, can produce both neuropathy and myopathy.[66] Morphologic evaluation of a muscle biopsy from a patient who had injudiciously taken this drug for a prolonged period of time showed scattered degenerating myofibers with aggregates of myelin figures, targetoid fibers, and rare necrotic myofibers (Fig. 7-15).

Emetine is an ipecac alkaloid used in the treatment of amebiasis and as an emetic. In addition to its well-known cardiotoxic effects, emetine may produce generalized skeletal muscle weakness when used excessively.[67-69] Clinically, the weakness resulting from emetine myopathy may simulate an inflammatory myopathy. The relatively few histologic studies that are available have shown foci of myofibrillar degeneration and internalization of myofiber nuclei. In contrast

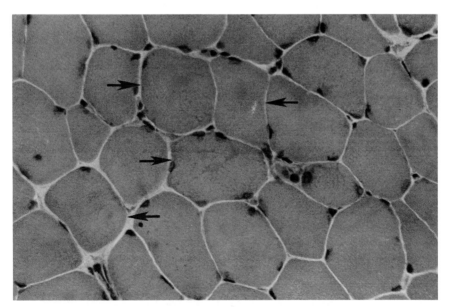

Figure 7-15. Muscle biopsy specimen from a 43-year-old woman who took colchicine injudiciously for a prolonged period of time. Note the targetoid fibers *(arrows)*. H&E, ×410.

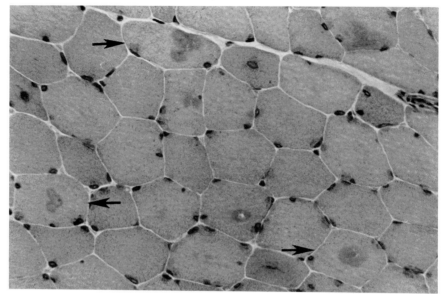

Figure 7-16. Muscle biopsy specimen from a 19-year-old woman with bulimia and ipecac abuse. Note the foci of myofibrillar disarray *(arrows)*. H&E, ×440.

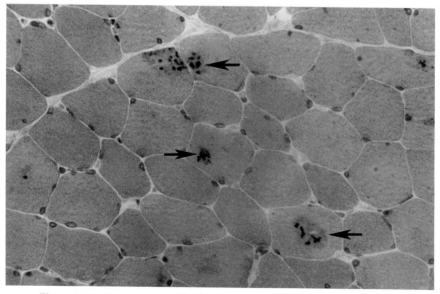

Figure 7-17. Emetine myopathy (same patient as in Fig. 7–16). Note the cytoplasmic bodies *(arrows)*. Trichrome, ×440.

to the inflammatory myopathies, there is no perifascicular atrophy, no interstitial inflammation, and only rare necrotic myofibers. The type I myofibers display targetoid changes and may contain multiple small corelike structures that resemble the alterations encountered in multicore disease. Internalized nuclei are encountered predominantly among the type I myofibers. The type II myofibers also may show myofibrillar derangements in the form of numerous cytoplasmic bodies (Figs. 7-16 and 7-17).

MALIGNANT HYPERTHERMIA

Malignant hyperthermia is a serious, potentially lethal syndrome that is most frequently precipitated by the administration of halogenated anesthetics and/or succinylcholine.[70] Susceptibility to the syndrome is thought to be inherited as an autosomal-dominant trait. Susceptible individuals do not necessarily develop symptoms upon exposure to these agents and nearly half of individuals at risk have had previous anesthesia without recognized disease. Symptoms, when they appear, vary in their rate of onset and severity. The clinical manifestations of the fully expressed syndrome include rapid rise in body temperature, tachycardia, cardiac arrhythmias, increased oxygen consumption, acidosis, muscle rigidity, disseminated intravascular coagulation, rhabdomyolysis, hyperkalemia, and renal failure. The disease is fatal in over 50 percent of the fully developed fulminant cases. The fundamental genetic abnormality responsible for this condition has not been elucidated, although the major metabolic derangement appears to be an increase in intracytoplasmic calcium. This leads to abnormal contractions and loss of metabolic control in muscle. Because of the potential risk of anesthesia, much effort has been made to identify susceptible individuals. In a few cases, malignant hyperthermia has been associated with central core disease or myotonic disorders.[71] Generally, routine histologic studies on muscle biopsy specimens from individuals known or suspected to be at risk for this disorder have shown only nonspecific alterations.[72] These include occasional atrophic myofibers, increased numbers of internal nuclei, and abnormal staining with oxidative enzyme stains such as the NADH–TR reaction. When present, the morphologic abnormalities seem to involve predominantly type I myofibers. Susceptibility to malignant hyperthermia *cannot* be diagnosed histologically. About two thirds of the patients at risk have increased serum CK levels. At the present time, however, the most reliable diagnostic test consists of in vitro study of muscle contraction upon exposure to caffeine and halothane.[70]

MYOADENYLATE DEAMINASE DEFICIENCY

Myoadenylate deaminase converts adenosine monophosphate to inosine monophosphate with the release of ammonia. Although the activity of this enzyme is greater in skeletal muscle than other tissues, the role of this enzyme in the normal metabolism of muscle is unestablished. It may be involved in the regulation of ATP level. Fishbein et al.[73] described deficient activity of this enzyme in five men with weakness and/or cramps induced by exercise. Subsequent studies have demonstrated this enzyme deficiency in other patients with exercise intolerance and in many other neuromuscular disorders.[74-76] The deficiency is common and has been observed in as many as 2 percent of muscle biopsy specimens. In normal muscle, the type I myofibers stain slightly bluer than the type II myofibers. Muscle specimens from patients with myoadenylate deaminase deficiency show little or no staining of either fiber type. The carrier state has been identified recently supporting an autosomal-recessive mode of inheritance.[77] Nevertheless, any relation between this enzyme deficiency and exercise intolerance or other neuromuscular disease remains unsettled.

MISCELLANEOUS METABOLIC DISEASES

There are various systemic metabolic diseases in which morphologic abnormalities can be demonstrated in skeletal muscle specimens even though involvement of skeletal muscle is not a prominent part of the disease process. This is especially true in the case of the neuronal ceroid lipofuscinoses. This is a group of closely related metabolic disorders that were formerly confused with the gangliosidoses, especially Tay-Sachs disease. The neuronal ceroid-lipofuscinoses are characterized by the accumulation of autofluorescent lipopigments in various tissues. The major clinical manifestations include varying degrees of mental retardation, seizures, and visual impairment. The syndrome can be divided into four relatively distinct types based on the age at the onset of these manifestations and the rate of disease progression.[78] The Haltia–Santavouri type is an infantile form characterized by very early onset of blindness and rapid neurologic deterioration but relatively few seizures. The late-infantile Jansky–Bielschowsky form usually begins with seizures between the ages of 2 and 5 years. The disease progresses rapidly, with severe seizures and marked mental deterioration. Visual impairment is a relatively late manifestation. The juvenile, Spielmeyer–Sjögren type generally begins somewhat later and is dominated by visual impairment. The adult form, Kufs' disease, progresses very slowly and is dominated by cerebellar and extrapyramidal signs. Mental deterioration is less severe than in the other types. Seizures and blindness are rare.

Although the clinical manifestations of this group of diseases reflect predominantly the involvement of the central nervous system and eyes, muscle specimens may be used for morphologic diagnosis. Frozen sections stained by the routine histochemical procedures, and paraffin-embedded sections generally show no evidence of abnormal lipopigment storage. Occasionally, examination with ultraviolet light will disclose abnormal deposits of autofluorescent material. Carpenter et al.[79] have also reported vacuoles that are partially filled with PAS-positive material that was resistant to digestion with diastase. Diagnostic features are more readily demonstrated by electron microscopy. Muscle from patients with the infantile (Haltia–Santavouri) type of neuronal ceroid lipofuscinosis harbor deposits of finely granular osmiophilic material (Fig. 7–18). In the late-infantile (Jansky–Bielschowsky) form, myofibers contain numerous membrane-bound deposits of curvilinear profiles beneath the sarcolemma (Fig. 7–19), and to a lesser extent between myofibrils.[80,81] Similar deposits may be found in the endothelial cells of intramuscular capillaries. In the juvenile (Spielmeyer–Sjögren) form, muscle fibers may contain deposits of identical curvilinear profiles[81] or cytosomes with so-called rectilinear profiles.[80] Curvilinear profiles have also been reported in muscle from patients with Kufs' disease.[82] Although electron microscopy of muscle biopsy specimens is an effective means of confirming a diagnosis of neuronal ceroid lipofuscinosis, it is not suitable for distinguishing among the various forms.

The biochemical defect responsible for neuronal ceroid lipofuscinosis has not been fully elucidated. Many workers regard the excessive accumulation of lipopigments to be the result of a genetically determined aberration in the control of intracellular peroxidation.[78] However, assays for myeloperoxidase deficiency are no longer regarded as significant or reliable for the diagnosis of

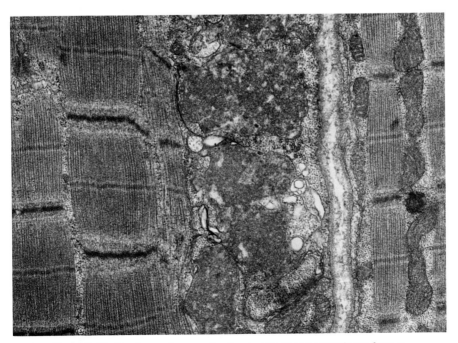

Figure 7-18. Electron micrograph of a muscle biopsy specimen from a child with the Haltia–Santavouri form of neuronal ceroid lipofuscinosis. Note the cytosomes containing finely granular osmiophilic material. ×27,000.

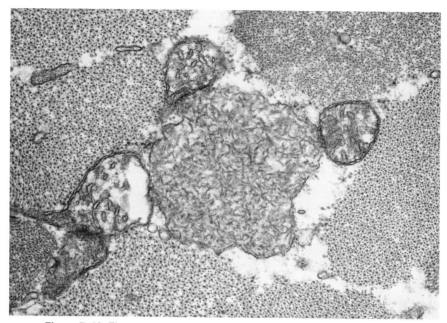

Figure 7-19. Electron micrograph of a muscle biopsy specimen from a child with the Jansky–Bielschowsky form of neuronal ceroid lipofuscinosis. Note the membrane-bound mass of curvilinear profiles. ×60,000.

these disorders.[83] Alternatively, some authors have suggested that the pigments result from storage of dolichols or retinoid-type complexes.[84,85]

Myoclonus epilepsy or Lafora's disease is a rare metabolic disease that affects predominantly the central nervous system. Clinically the disease is characterized by the onset of seizures and myoclonus during adolescence. The patients undergo personality changes, become demented, and often die within 5 to 10 years. Histologically, the disease is characterized by the presence of Lafora bodies. These spherical inclusion bodies are found within the perikarya and processes of neurons throughout the cerebral cortex and basal ganglia. They are especially numerous in the substantia nigra and dentate nucleus. They are basophilic or amphophilic with H&E and are strongly PAS-positive. Ultrastructurally, they consist of unbounded masses of granular and fibrillar material. These have been shown to consist of polyglucosans.

Patients with myoclonus epilepsy may have polyglucosan deposits in liver, skin, myocardium, and skeletal muscle. The deposits in skeletal muscle are relatively inconspicuous and inconsistently encountered. By light microscopy, they appear as fine PAS-positive granules[86,87] By electron microscopy, the deposits consist of granular and fibrillar material. Unfortunately, skeletal muscle is not a reliable tissue for the morphologic diagnosis of this disease.

References

1. DiMauro S: Metabolic myopathies. In Vinken PJ, Bruyn GW (eds): Handbook of Clinical Neurology. Amsterdam, North-Holland, 1979, Vol 41, pp 175–234.
2. Essen B, Jansson E, Henriksson J, et al.: Metabolic characteristics of fibre types in human skeletal muscle. Acta Physiol Scand 95:153–165, 1975.
3. Bradley WG, Hudgson P, Gardner-Medwin D, Walton JN: Myopathy associated with abnormal lipid metabolism in skeletal muscle. Lancet 1:495–498, 1969.
4. Engel WK, Vick NA, Glueck J, Levy RI: A skeletal muscle disorder associated with intermittent symptoms and possible defect in lipid metabolism. N Engl J Med 282:697–704, 1970.
5. Engel AG, Angelini C: Carnitine deficiency of human skeletal muscle with associated lipid myopathy: A new syndrome. Science 179:899–901, 1973.
6. Bradley WG, Jenkison M, Park DC, et al.: A myopathy associated with lipid storage. J Neurol Sci 16:137–154, 1972.
7. Isaacs H, Heffron JJA, Badenhorst M, Pickering A: Weakness associated with the pathological presence of lipid in skeletal muscle: A detailed study of a patient with carnitine deficiency. J Neurol Neurosurg Psychiatry 39:1114–1123, 1976.
8. Markesbery WR, McQuillen MP, Procopis PG, et al.: Muscle carnitine deficiency. Arch Neurol 31:320–324, 1974.
9. Karpati G, Carpenter S, Engel AG, et al.: The syndrome of systemic carnitine deficiency. Neurology 25:16–24, 1975.
10. Chapoy PR, Angelini C, Brown WJ, et al.: Systemic carnitine deficiency—A treatable inherited lipid-storage disease presenting as Reye's syndrome. N Engl J Med 303:1389–1394, 1980.
11. Tripp ME, Katcher ML, Peters HA, et al.: Systemic carnitine deficiency presenting as familial endocardial fibroelastosis. N Engl J Med 305:385–390, 1981.
12. Carroll JE, Brooke MH, DeVivo DC, et al.: Carnitine "deficiency": Lack of response to carnitine therapy. Neurology 30:608–626, 1980.
13. Boudin G, Mikol J, Guillard A, Engel AG: Fatal systemic carnitine deficiency with lipid storage in skeletal muscle, heart, liver and kidney. J Neurol Sci 30:313–325, 1976.
14. Engel AG, Banker BQ, Eiben RM: Carnitine deficiency: Clinical, morphological, and biochemical observations in a fatal case. J Neurol Neurosurg Psychiatry 40:313–322, 1977.
15. Rebouche CJ, Engel AG: Primary systemic carnitine deficiency. I. Carnitine biosynthesis. Neurology 31:813–818, 1981.
16. Engel AG, Rebouche CJ, Wilson DM, et al.: Primary systemic carnitine deficiency. II. Renal handling of carnitine. Neurology 31:819–825, 1981.
17. DiMauro S, Trevisan C, Hays A: Disorders of lipid metabolism in muscle. Muscle Nerve 3:369–388, 1980.
18. McComas CF, Riggs JE, Breen LA, et al.: Neurologic complications following gastric plication. Neurology 33 (Suppl 2):191, 1980.
19. DiMauro S, DiMauro PMM: Muscle carnitine palmityltransferase deficiency and myoglobinuria. Science 182:929–931, 1973.
20. Miranda A, DiMauro S, Eastwood A, et al.: Lipid storage, myopathy, ichthyosis, and steatorrhea. Muscle Nerve 2:1–13, 1979.
21. Angelini C, Philippart M, Borrone C, et al.: Multisystem triglyceride storage disorder with impaired long-chain fatty acid oxidation. Ann Neurol 7:5–10, 1980.

22. Jerusalem F, Spiess H, Baumgartner G: Lipid storage myopathy with normal carnitine levels. J Neurol Sci 24:273–282, 1975.

23. Jerusalem F, Angelini C, Engel AG, Groover RV: Mitochondria–lipid–glycogen (MLG) disease of muscle. Arch Neurol 29:162–169, 1973.

24. Askanas V, Engel WK, Kwan HH, et al.: Autosomal dominant syndrome of lipid neuromyopathy with normal carnitine: Successful treatment with long-chain fatty-acid-free diet. Neurology 35:66–72, 1985.

25. Sarnat HB, Roth SI, Carroll JE, et al.: Lipid storage in infantile Pompe's disease. Arch Neurol 39:180–183, 1982.

26. Engel AG: Acid maltase deficiency in adults: Studies in four cases of a syndrome which may mimic muscular dystrophy or other myopathies. Brain 93:599–616, 1970.

27. Luft R, Ikkos D, Palmieri G, et al.: A case of severe hypermetabolism of nonthyroid origin with a defect in the maintenance of mitochondrial respiratory control: A correlated clinical, biochemical and morphological study. J Clin Invest 41:1776–1804, 1962.

28. Afifi AK, Ibrahim MZB, Bergman RA, et al.: Morphologic features of hypermetabolic mitochondrial disease: A light microscopic, histochemical and electron microscopic study. J Neurol Sci 15:271–290, 1972.

29. DiMauro S, Bonilla E, Lee CP, et al.: Luft's disease: Further biochemical and ultrastructural studies of skeletal muscle in the second case. J Neurol Sci 27:217–232, 1976.

30. Shy GM, Gonatas NK: Human myopathy with giant abnormal mitochondria. Science 145:493–496, 1964.

31. Shy GM, Gonatas NK, Perez M: Two childhood myopathies with abnormal mitochondria. I. Megaconial myopathy. II. Pleoconial myopathy. Brain 89:133–158, 1966.

32. Morgan-Hughes JA: Mitochondrial myopathies. In Mastaglia FL, Walton J (eds): Skeletal Muscle Pathology. Edinburgh, Churchill Livingstone, 1982, pp 309–339.

33. Olson W, Engel WK, Walsh GO, Einaugler R: Oculocraniosomatic neuromuscular disease with "ragged-red" fibers. Arch Neurol 26:193–211, 1972.

34. Bonilla E, Schotland DL, DiMauro S, Aldover B: Electron cytochemistry of crystalline inclusions in human skeletal muscle mitochondria. J Ultrastruct Res 51:404–408, 1975.

35. Melmed C, Karpati G, Carpenter S: Experimental mitochondrial myopathy produced by in vitro uncoupling of oxidative phosphorylation. J Neurol Sci 26:305–318, 1975.

36. Carpenter S, Karpati G: Pathology of Skeletal Muscle. New York, Churchill Livingstone, 1984, pp. 604–605.

37. Blass JP: Disorders of pyruvate metabolism. Neurology 29:280–286, 1979.

38. Crosby TW, Chou SM: "Ragged-red" fibers in Leigh's disease. Neurology 24:49–54, 1974.

39. Riggs JE, Schochet SS Jr, Fakadej AV, et al.: Mitochondrial encephalomyopathy with decreased succinate–cytochrome c reductase activity. Neurology 34:48–53, 1984.

40. DiMauro S, Mendell JR, Sahenk Z, et al.: Fatal infantile mitochondrial myopathy and renal dysfunction due to cytochrome-c-oxidase deficiency. Neurology 30:795–804, 1980.

41. Karpati G, Carpenter S, Larbrisseau A, Lafontaine R: The Kearns–Shy syndrome. A multisystem disease with mitochondrial abnormalities demonstrated in skeletal muscle and skin. J Neurol Sci 19:133–151, 1973.

42. Berenberg RA, Pellock JM, DiMauro S, et al.: Lumping or splitting? "Ophthalmoplegia-plus" or Kearns–Sayre syndrome. Ann Neurol 1:37–54, 1977.

43. Coulter DL, Allen RJ: Abrupt neurological deterioration in children with Kearns–Sayre syndrome. Arch Neurol 38:247–250, 1981.

44. Gonatas NK, Evangelista I, Martin J: A generalized disorder of nervous system, skeletal muscle and heart resembling Refsum's disease and Hurler's syndrome. II. Ultrastructure. Am J Med 42:169–178, 1967.

45. Adachi M, Torii J, Volk BW, et al.: Electron microscopic and enzyme histochemical studies of cerebellum, ocular and skeletal muscles in chronic progressive ophthalmoplegia with cerebellar ataxia. Acta Neuropathol 23:300–312, 1973.

46. Mitsumoto H, Aprille JR, Wray SH, et al.: Chronic progressive external ophthalmoplegia (CPED): Clinical, morphologic, and biochemical studies. Neurology 33:452–461, 1983.

47. Harriman DGF, Reed R: The incidence of lipid droplets in human skeletal muscular disorders: A histochemical, electron microscopic and freeze-etch study. J Pathol 106:1–24, 1972.

48. Engel AG: Electron microscopic observations in thyrotoxic and corticosteroid-induced myopathies. Mayo Clin Proc 41:785–796, 1966.

49. Schutta HS, Armitage JL: Thyrotoxic hypokalemic periodic paralysis. A fine structure study. J Neuropathol Exp Neurol 28:321–336, 1969.

50. Ewing SL, Rosai J: Basophilic (mucoid) degeneration of skeletal muscle. Arch Pathol 97:60–62, 1974.

51. Ho KL: Basophilic degeneration of skeletal muscle in hypothyroid myopathy. Arch Pathol Lab Med 108:239–245, 1984.

52. Patten BM, Bilezikian JP, Mallette LE, et al.: Neuromuscular disease in primary hyperparathyroidism. Ann Intern Med 80:182–193, 1974.

53. Britt CW, Light RR, Peters BH, Schochet SS Jr: Rhabdomyolysis during treatment with epsilon-aminocaproic acid. Arch Neurol 37:187–188, 1980.

54. Penn AS: Myoglobin and myoglobinuria. In Vinken PJ, Bruyn GW (eds): Handbook of Clinical Neurology. Amsterdam, North-Holland, 1979, Vol 41, pp 259–285.

55. Geller SA: Extreme exertion rhabdomyolysis. A histopathologic study of 31 cases. Hum Pathol 4:241–250, 1973.

56. Adams RD: Traumatic necrosis of pretibial muscles (anterior tibial syndrome). In Diseases of Muscle. A study in Pathology, 3rd ed. Hagerstown, Md., Harper & Row, 1975, pp 405–408.

57. Schmitt HP, Bersch W, Feustel HP: Acute abdominal rhabdomyolysis after body building exercise: Is there a "rectus abdominis syndrome?" Muscle Nerve 6:228–232, 1983.

58. Gabow PA, Kaehny WD, Kelleher SP: The spectrum of rhabdomyolysis. Medicine 61:141–152, 1982.

59. Rubenstein AE, Wainapel SF: Acute hypokalemic myopathy in alcoholism. Arch Neurol 34:553–555, 1977.

60. Chui LA, Neustein H, Munsat TL: Tubular aggregates in subclinical alcoholic myopathy. Neurology 25:405–412, 1975.

61. Gamboa ET, Eastwood AB, Hays AP, et al.: Isolation of influenza virus from muscle in myoglobinuric polymyositis. Neurology 29:1323–1335, 1979.

62. Whisnant JP, Espinosa RE, Kierland RR, Lambert EH: Chloroquine neuromyopathy. Mayo Clin Proc 38:501–513, 1963.

63. Itabashi HH, Kokmen E: Chloroquine neuromyopathy. A reversible granulovacuolar myopathy. Arch Pathol 93:209–218, 1972.

64. MacDonald RD, Engel AG: Experimental chloroquine myopathy. J Neuropathol Exp Neurol 29:479–499, 1970.

65. Neville HE, Maunder-Sewry CA, McDougall J, et al.: Chloroquine-induced cytosomes with curvilinear profiles in muscle. Muscle Nerve 2:376–381, 1979.

66. Kontos HA: Myopathy associated with chronic colchicine toxicity. N Engl J Med 266:38–39, 1962.

67. Bennett HS, Spiro AJ, Pollack MA, Zucker P: Ipecac-induced myopathy simulating dermatomyositis. Neurology 32:91–94, 1982.

68. Sugie H, Russin R, Verity MA: Emetine myopathy: Two case reports with pathobiochemical analysis. Muscle Nerve 7:54–59, 1984.

69. Mateer JE, Farrell BJ, Chou SM, Gutmann L: Reversible ipecac myopathy. Arch Neurol 42:188–190, 1985.

70. Nelson TE, Flewellen EH: The malignant hyperthermia syndrome. N Engl J Med 309:416–418, 1983.

71. Eng GD, Epstein BS, Engel WEK, et al.: Malignant hyperthermia and central core disease in a child with congenital dislocating hips. Arch Neurol 35:189–197, 1978.

72. Harriman DGF: The pathology of malignant hyperpyrexia. In Mastaglia FL, Walton J (eds): Skeletal Muscle Pathology. Edinburgh, Churchill Livingstone, 1982, pp 575–591.

73. Fishbein WN, Armbrustmacher VW, Griffin JL: Myoadenylate deaminase deficiency: A new disease of muscle. Science 200:545–548, 1978.

74. Shumate JB, Katnik R, Ruiz M, et al.: Myoadenylate deaminase deficiency. Muscle Nerve 2:213–216, 1979.

75. Kar NC, Pearson CM: Muscle adenylate deaminase deficiency: Report of six new cases. Arch Neurol 38:279–281, 1981.

76. Keleman J, Rice DR, Bradley WG, et al.: Familial myoadenylate deaminase deficiency and exertional myalgia. Neurology 32:857–863, 1982.

77. Fishbein WN, Armbrustmacher VW, Griffin JL, et al.: Levels of adenylate deaminase, adenylate kinase and creatine kinase in frozen human muscle biopsy specimens relative to type 1/type 2 fiber distribution: Evidence for a carrier state of myoadenylate deaminase deficiency. Ann Neurol 15:271–277, 1984.

78. Zeman W: The neuronal ceroid lipofuscinoses. Prog Neuropathol 3:203–223, 1976.

79. Carpenter S, Karpati G, Wolfe LS, Andermann F: A type of juvenile cerebromacular degeneration characterized by granular osmiophilic deposits. J Neurol Sci 18:67–87, 1973.

80. Carpenter S, Karpati G, Andermann F: Specific involvement of muscle, nerve, and skin in late infantile and juvenile amaurotic idiocy. Neurology 22:170–186, 1972.

81. Goebel HH, Zeman W, Pilz H: Significance of muscle biopsies in neuronal ceroid-lipofuscinoses. J Neurol Neurosurg Psychiatry 38:985–993, 1975.

82. Dom R, Brucher JM, Ceuterick C, et al.: Adult ceroid-lipofuscinosis (Kufs' disease) in two brothers. Retinal and visceral storage in one; diagnostic muscle biopsy in the other. Acta Neuropathol 45:67–72, 1979.

83. Pilz H, Schwendermann G, Goebel HH: Diagnostic significance of myeloperoxidase assay in neuronal ceroid-lipofuscinoses (Batten–Vogt syndrome). Neurology 28:924–927, 1978.

84. Wolfe LS, Ng Ying Kin NMK, Baker RR, et al.: Identification of retinoyl complexes as the autofluorescent component of the neuronal storage material in Batten disease. Science 195:1360–1362, 1977.

85. Wolfe LS, Ng Ying Kin NMK, Palo J, Haltia M: Dolichols in brain and urinary sediment in neuronal ceroid lipofuscinosis. Neurology 33:103–106, 1983.
86. Carpenter S, Karpati G, Andermann F, et al.: Lafora's disease: Peroxisomal storage in skeletal muscle. Neurology 24:531–538, 1974.
87. Neville HE, Brooke MH, Austin JH: Studies in myoclonus epilepsy (Lafora body form). IV. Skeletal muscle abnormalities. Arch Neurol 30:466–474, 1974.

chapter 8

Congenital Myopathies

The so-called "congenital myopathies" are a large, heterogeneous group of disorders with overlapping clinical manifestations. Most have been delineated on the basis of relatively characteristic morphologic features. The designation "congenital myopathy" is somewhat of a misnomer. Despite the common usage of the term, there is considerable disagreement as to whether these diseases are truly developmental myopathies or whether they are the result of aberrant innervation. Furthermore, there is considerable variation in the age of presentation. Although these diseases may become apparent in early infancy, causing the "floppy infant" syndrome, in other patients the diseases do not become apparent until later in childhood or even adult life. The clinical course of individuals with these disorders are varied. Many infants with these diseases have a relatively benign course, with the weakness and hypotonia remaining static or improving. Other patients, however, have a rapidly progressive course leading to an early demise, often from respiratory complications. When encountered in older individuals, the diseases may have been nearly asymptomatic or may have pursued a progressive course. In many childhood cases the muscular weakness and hypotonia are accompanied by skeletal anomalies such as high arched palate, pectus excavatum, kyphoscoliosis, and dislocated hips.

For the most part, these conditions cannot be distinguished from one another clinically. Electromyography generally shows only nonspecific changes. Serum muscle enzymes are generally normal or only mildly elevated. The diagnosis of these conditions is based largely on morphologic features demonstrated in muscle biopsy specimens. In addition to histologic alterations that are considered characteristic for each of these individual diseases, there are other morphologic findings that are common to many of these entities. The latter include type I myofiber predominance and often a relatively small size of the type I myofibers. Brooke et al.[1] have suggested that in the infantile cases the clinical manifestations may parallel the type I myofiber predominance more closely than the specific architectural changes in the myofibers.

In addition to the well-documented forms of congenital myopathy, there are other disorders that have been encountered in only a single or very few cases. The discussions that follow will include only some of the more common and better documented entities.

CENTRAL CORE DISEASE

Central core disease was the first of the morphologically distinctive congenital myopathies to be clearly delineated. In 1956, Shy and Magee[2] reported the occurrence of weakness, hypotonia, and abnormal posturing in five patients from three generations of a single family. At the time of their report, the patients ranged in age from 2 to 65 years. Subsequently, many more cases have been reported, confirming and expanding the original observations. Infants with this disease may present with the "floppy infant" syndrome. Children may have weakness, hypotonia, and delayed motor development. In these patients, skeletal anomalies including short stature, kyphoscoliosis, congenitally dislocated hips, and pes cavus are frequently encountered.[3] Adults with central core disease may show varying degrees of proximal muscular weakness that is more pronounced in the lower limbs. Occasionally, the morphologic features of this disease have been found in adults who are nearly asymptomatic. A further concern is the fact that the malignant hyperthermia syndrome has occurred in some families with central core disease.[4] Many of the patients, including the ones in the family originally described by Shy and Magee,[2] appear to have inherited the disease as an autosomal-dominant trait. Other cases are apparently sporadic.

The disorder was designated as central core disease because of the characteristic appearance of the abnormal myofibers. The interior of the affected myofibers contain one or more cylindrical structures, the so-called cores. These extend for a considerable distance, probably throughout the entire length of the myofiber. The cores are more readily seen in cross-section.

Cores can be demonstrated readily in frozen sections with a wide variety of stains. With H&E and the modified trichrome procedures, they generally appear more homogeneous than the periphery of the myofiber (Figs. 8-1 and 8-2). Occasionally the cores are more clearly demarcated by a dark-staining line or band (Fig. 8-3). With PAS and myophosphorylase techniques, the cores display reduced staining. Generally they are most clearly demonstrated with the NADH–TR stain (Fig. 8-4). With this technique, the cores are unstained and stand in striking contrast to the darkly stained periphery of the myofiber. Cores also may be demonstrated with the nonspecific esterase technique in which case they stain more darkly than the surrounding intact portion of the myofiber.

The cores are inconspicuous or even appear as "negative images" with the ATPase techniques (Fig. 8-5). Nevertheless, these stains vividly demonstrate other histologic characteristics of the disease. Although the percentage of fibers containing cores varies from patient to patient, the cores are restricted to type I myofibers. Furthermore, most cases show type I myofiber predominance. In

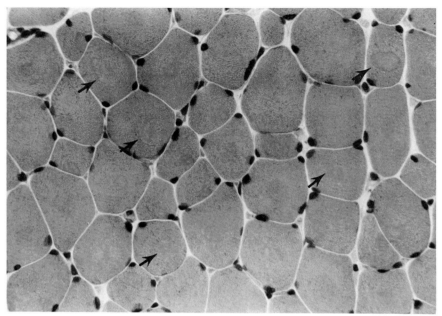

Figure 8-1. Central core disease in a 20-year-old woman with a lifelong history of mild proximal muscle weakness. Numerous myofibers contain central cores *(arrows)*. Although the cores stain a similar color, they are more homogeneous than the surrounding sarcoplasm. H&E, ×420.

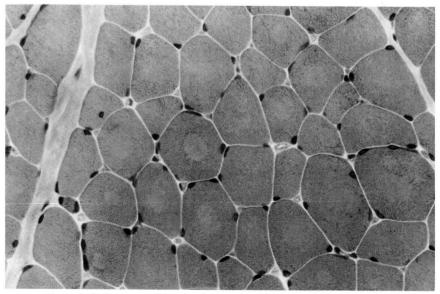

Figure 8-2. Central core disease, same patient as in Figure 8-1. Trichrome, ×420.

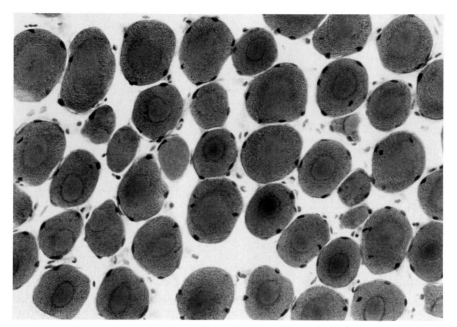

Figure 8-3. Central core disease in an 8½-year-old girl. Both this girl and her mother had proximal muscle weakness that was most marked in the lower limbs. In this patient, the cores are clearly demarcated by a darker-staining band between the core and surrounding sarcoplasm. Trichrome, ×340.

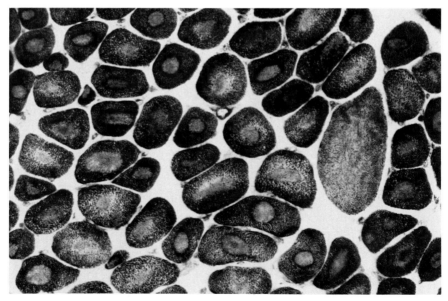

Figure 8-4. Central core disease, same patient as in Figure 8-3. The cores are generally best seen with the NADH-TR reaction. ×320.

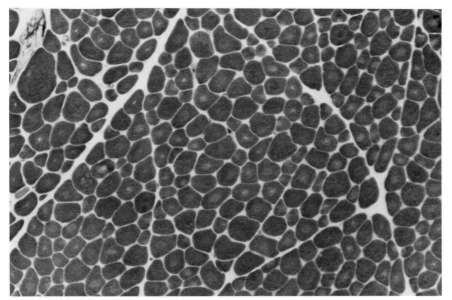

Figure 8-5. Another characteristic feature of central core disease is type I myofiber predominance. Virtually all the myofibers are stained uniformly darkly. ATPase following preincubation at pH 4.3, × 175.

some specimens, virtually all of the myofibers appear to be type I myofibers. This important feature helps in distinguishing central core disease from disorders with florid target fiber formation.

Although less consistently reliable, cores often can be demonstrated in paraffin-embedded sections. In fact, the morphologic descriptions in the original report of this disease were derived predominantly from paraffin-embedded sections.[2] The cores were seen with H&E but were more clearly delineated with a trichrome stain that colored the cores blue in contrast to the red of the surrounding portions of the myofibers. In addition to these stains, PTAH also can be used effectively on paraffin-embedded sections (Fig. 8-6). The extent to which cores retain their sarcomeric periodicity varies and has been the subject of conflicting reports. In the cases reported by Shy and Magee,[2] examination by phase microscopy and with polarized light disclosed striations within the cores. This has not been a consistent finding in subsequent cases. Neville and Brooke[5] investigated cores by electron microscopy and described two types, structured and unstructured. The myofibrils within the structured cores were well organized and retained sarcomeric periodicity. The sarcomeres, however, were shorter and were out of register with the periphery of the myofiber. By contrast, the myofibrils within the unstructured cores were extensively disorganized and showed Z-disc streaming. Thus the unstructured cores closely resemble target fibers. Both types of cores lacked mitochondria and contained reduced quantities of glycogen and sarcoplasmic reticulum. These findings cor-

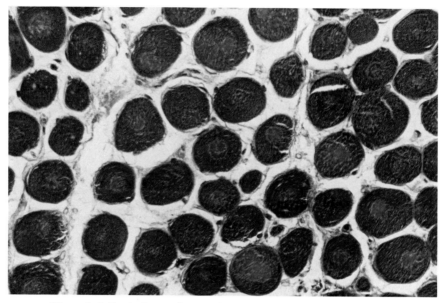

Figure 8–6. Central core disease. In many patients, the cores can be seen in paraffin-embedded sections. PTAH, ×420.

relate with the reduced NADH–TR, phosphorylase, and PAS staining demonstrated histochemically. In some patients, cores of both types have been encountered concurrently.[3] Most of the specimens that we have examined have contained predominantly unstructured cores. Rarely, nemaline rods have been encountered in association with cores, and in biopsy specimens from other family members of patients with central core disease.[6]

The pathogenetic mechanisms for core formation are unknown. Because of the similarities between target fibers and cores, some authors have suggested that central core disease is the result of aberrant innervation. Furthermore, Telerman-Toppet et al.[3] observed an increased innervation ratio suggesting reinnervation. However, studies with alpha-bungarotoxin have failed to show increased extrajunctional acetylcholine receptor activity, as would be expected following denervation.[7] Myofiber structural changes somewhat resembling cores have been produced experimentally in animals by tenotomy.[8] There are still substantial differences, however, between the experimental lesions and naturally occurring cores and target fibers.[9]

MULTICORE DISEASE

Multicore disease was defined by Engel et al.[10] as a congenital, nonprogressive myopathy characterized by the presence of numerous small foci of myofibrillary degeneration. The original patients had weakness of trunk and proximal limb muscles, reduced muscle bulk, and delayed motor development. The clinical spectrum has been expanded by additional publications. Heffner et al.[11] reported the disease in twin boys with torticollis. These cases, along with three siblings reported by Dubowitz,[12] suggest that the disease may be inherited as an autosomal-recessive trait. Bonnette et al.[13] described a progressive form of this disorder with onset of the clinical manifestations during adulthood.

Morphologically, multicore disease is characterized by numerous fusiform areas in which there is loss of striations and abnormal myofiber staining. The same lesions have been described by the somewhat more descriptive term "minicores."[12] The abnormal foci are most clearly demonstrated with the NADH–TR reaction since they show reduced oxidative enzyme reactivity. They can also be seen with the myophosphorylase and ATPase techniques. The multicore lesions are typically found in type I myofibers that are somewhat smaller than normal and smaller than the accompanying type II myofibers. The specimens also show type I myofiber predominance. Internal nuclei may be mildly increased in number. By electron microscopy, the lesions are characterized by a reduced number of mitochondria, myofibrillar disorganization, and Z-disc streaming. In contrast to central cores, the multicore lesions are smaller, more numerous, and often oriented perpendicular to the long axis of the myofiber.

NEMALINE MYOPATHY

Nemaline myopathy is characterized by the presence of small rod-shaped structures in affected myofibers. This disease, in the form of a congenital myopathy, was described independently by two different groups of investigators in 1963. Conen et al.[14] reported the disease in a weak, hypotonic child. They described the distinctive morphologic abnormality as "myogranules." Shy et al.[15] reported this morphologically distinctive disease in a 4-year-old boy. A muscle biopsy specimen from his clinically affected mother showed no morphologic changes. A muscle biopsy specimen from his father showed abnormalities of fiber size but no nemaline rods. An affected brother was not biopsied. Shy et al.[15] called the disease "nemaline myopathy." They chose this name since they thought that the morphologically unique bodies "could represent rods or coils of thread-like fibrous structure." Furthermore, they suggested that the disease might be inherited as an autosomal-dominant trait with variable expressivity.

Subsequent reports have expanded the spectrum of clinical manifestations associated with this disorder. A few patients with severe weakness and hypotonia as neonates have a rapidly progressive course and die of respiratory complications early in infancy.[16-18] More commonly, children with this disease have a more "benign," nonprogressive course despite weakness, hypotonia, and delayed motor development. Many have skeletal abnormalities including a narrow face, high arched palate, kyphoscoliosis, and clubbed feet. The weakness tends to be more severe proximally than distally but is often less severe than suggested by the reduced muscle bulk. Facial, palatal, and pharyngeal muscles may be affected but the extraocular muscles are spared. Rarely, the disease is first detected in adult life. Here too there is a wide spectrum of severity. Some individuals are asymptomatic, others have mild weakness dating from childhood, while still others manifest progressive disease.[19-24] Some of the adults have prominent wasting of distal leg muscles.[19,21,22] Other adults with progressive disease have additional histologic features not commonly encountered in the childhood cases. Engel and Oberc[20] reported the occurrence of nemaline rods in myofiber nuclei as well as among the contractile elements. This has been seen only once among the infantile cases.[25] Cardiac muscle is generally thought to be spared in cases of nemaline myopathy. Nevertheless, Meier et al.[26] recently reported a young adult who presented clinically with a cardiomyopathy. Histologic studies revealed typical changes of nemaline myopathy in skeletal muscle and numerous nemaline rods in the myocardium.

A wide variety of genetic patterns have been suggested for the inheritance of nemaline myopathy. Kondo and Yuasa[27] analyzed family patterns from 50 patients and concluded that the disease is probably inherited as an autosomal-dominant trait with reduced penetrance. The preponderance of females among the reported cases has led to the alternative suggestion that the disease might be inherited as an X-linked dominant trait that is semilethal in males.[28] Other authors have variously considered their cases to be sporadic or autosomal-recessive.

Diagnosis of this condition is based almost entirely on morphologic demonstration of the characteristic nemaline rods in skeletal muscle. Serum muscle enzymes are usually normal. Electromyography generally shows no abnormalities or only nonspecific myopathic changes. The nemaline rods are often difficult to detect in paraffin-embedded sections. Only rarely can they be seen in paraffin-embedded tissue stained with H&E. They are more readily seen in paraffin sections stained by PTAH or when viewed by phase microscopy.

As with many muscle diseases, frozen sections are more suitable for investigating this disease. Nemaline rods are most readily demonstrated with the modified trichrome procedure. With this stain, the rods appear as reddish-purple granules, 2 to 7 μm in diameter, that stand in contrast to the green of the myofiber (Figs. 8-7 and 8-8). Although the individual nemaline rods are quite small, they may be very conspicuous since they tend to occur in groups. They are often aggregated beneath the sarcolemma in one portion of the myofiber. The number of rods and number of fibers containing rods vary greatly from patient to patient and even among different muscles in the same patient (Fig. 8-9). There seems to be little or no correlation between the number of rods and the severity of the disease. The nemaline rods are not well demonstrated with the oxidative enzyme or ATPase stains. However, these techniques show three additional features of the disease. Rods are found predominantly if not exclusively in type I myofibers, the myofibers are often abnormally small, and there is a variable degree of type I myofiber predominance. In some patients the degree of fiber-type predominance varies from fascicle to fascicle, while in other patients almost no type II myofibers can be identified. It has

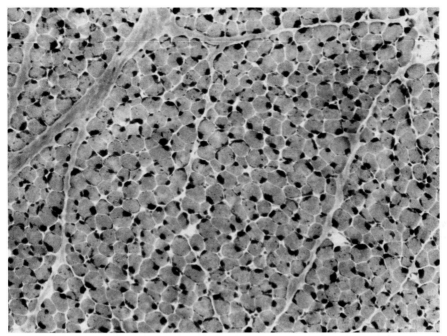

Figure 8-7. Nemaline myopathy in a 4-year-old boy with severe muscle weakness and mild skeletal anomalies. A large proportion of the myofibers in this patient contain deposits of nemaline rods. The deposits have a reddish color. Trichrome, × 175.

been suggested that the alterations in the size and proportion of type I myofibers may correlate more closely with the clinical manifestations of the disease than the presence or absence of rods.[1] However, type I myofiber predominance has been observed in clinically asymptomatic relatives of patients with nemaline myopathy.[28] In a few cases, nemaline rods have been encountered concurrently with morphologic features of other congenital myopathies. Karpati et al.[29] described the presence of central cores in a patient with nemaline myopathy and Afifi et al.[6] described these two alterations in different members of a single family. Muscle spindles are generally free of nemaline rods although involvement of intrafusal fibers has been reported occasionally.[16]

When abundant, the nemaline rods can be demonstrated very dramatically in epoxy sections stained by simple techniques such as alkaline toluidine blue (Fig. 8-10). By electron microscopy, the nemaline rods appear as elongated osmiophilic structures that are in continuity with the Z-discs.[30] In longitudinal sections, they appear to consist of compactly aggregated parallel filaments with periodic cross-striations at intervals of about 17 nm (Fig. 8-11). At their free ends, the rods appear to be in continuity with the thin myofilaments. In transverse sections, nemaline rods display a quadratic latticework configuration that

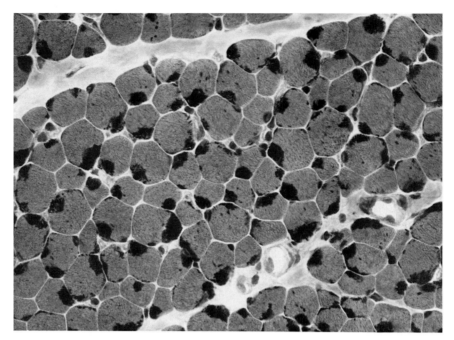

Figure 8-8. Nemaline myopathy, same patient as in Figure 8-7. At higher magnification, the granular nature of the deposits becomes apparent. Trichrome, ×500.

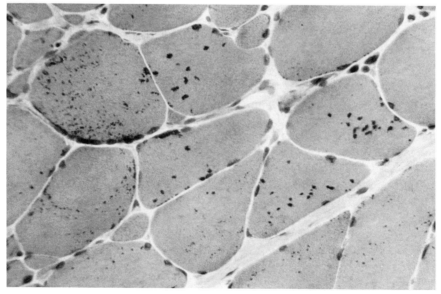

Figure 8-9. Biopsy specimens from other patients with nemaline myopathy, such as this 34-year-old woman, disclose only a relatively small number of nemaline rods. Trichrome, ×420.

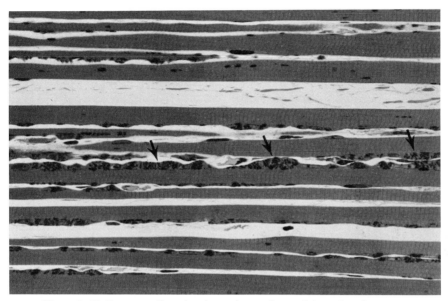

Figure 8-10. Epoxy section showing subsarcolemmal deposits of nemaline rods *(arrows).* Toluidine blue, ×500.

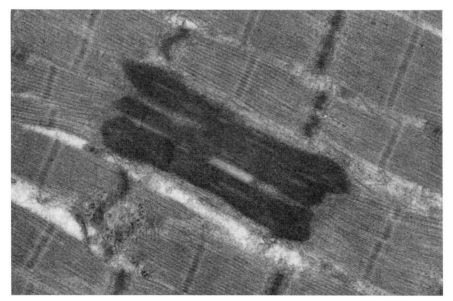

Figure 8-11. By electron microscopy, nemaline rods appear as elongated structures composed of compactly aggregated parallel filaments with periodic cross-striations. ×40,000.

is very similar to comparably sectioned Z-discs. The lattice squares each measure approximately 10 nm and appear to be formed by filaments that measure approximately 3 nm in diameter.

Although nemaline rods have been the subject of intense investigation, their precise composition and pathogenesis remains unsettled. Biochemical and immunohistochemical studies suggest that they contain predominantly alpha-actinin.[31] A defect in the control mechanisms that normally restrict alpha-actinin to the Z-discs in skeletal muscle has been proposed as the mechanism responsible for the formation of nemaline rods.[32]

Although the presence of nemaline rods is the hallmark of nemaline myopathy, these structures are not entirely disease specific. Occasional nemaline rods, usually in association with other myofiber abnormalities, have been observed in a wide variety of neuromuscular disorders. These include muscular dystrophies, myotonic dystrophy, and inflammatory myopathies. They also may be seen near myotendinous insertions and in the extraocular muscles of normal individuals.[33] They have been produced experimentally in animals by tenotomy.[8]

CENTRONUCLEAR MYOPATHY

The disease, or more correctly, the syndrome now commonly designated as either centronuclear myopathy or myotubular myopathy was originally described in 1966 by Spiro et al.[34] These authors reported a 12-year-old boy with a lifelong history of weakness and impaired motor development. The weakness involved extraocular and facial muscles as well as muscles of the trunk and extremities. Muscle biopsy specimens disclosed centrally located nuclei in a large proportion of the myofibers. The abnormal muscle fibers were thought to result from arrested development of the fetal myotubes and the disorder was termed "myotubular myopathy." Shortly thereafter, Sher et al.[35] reported two sisters, aged 18 and 16 years, who had impaired motor development and diffuse weakness including weakness of the extraocular muscles. One also had weakness of facial muscles. Muscle biopsy specimens from these two girls disclosed relatively small myofibers with a very high proportion of centrally located nuclei. Although the patients' mother was asymptomatic except for mild ptosis, biopsy specimen showed increased variation in myofiber size and centrally located nuclei in a large proportion of the myofibers, especially the smaller myofibers. Sher et al.[35] designated this condition as "centronuclear myopathy" and suggested that it was transmitted as an autosomal-dominant trait.

Although the patients described in these original reports had rather similar clinical features, subsequent reports greatly expanded the clinical spectrum and suggested additional patterns of transmission for the disorder.[36] At the present time, at least three more or less distinct categories can be delineated. Some patients, with onset of symptoms as neonates, have a very pernicious course leading to death from respiratory complications at any early age. This form of the disorder was originally described in two unrelated Dutch families in which it was transmitted as an X-linked recessive trait.[37,38] Paraffin-embedded sections from the deceased males showed a mixture of normal-appearing fibers and abnormally small, hollow, "myotubelike" fibers with centrally located nuclei. Engel et al.[39] described under the designation of "type I fiber hypotrophy and central nuclei" a hypotonic male infant who died of respiratory complications at 18 months of age. Histologically, this patient was characterized by strikingly small type I myofibers and internal nuclei in about 25 percent of small myofibers, regardless of type. Some authors regard this case as another example of myotubular myopathy with neonatal onset and relatively rapid progression. Other patients, however, with onset of symptoms as neonates and the same histologic findings, have a more benign course.[12]

In most cases of centronuclear myopathy, the manifestations of the disease become apparent during early childhood or late infancy.[36,40–42] As in other congenital myopathies, the children are often weak, hypotonic, and have delayed motor development. Weakness of the extraocular muscles is often the only clinical feature suggestive of the specific diagnosis. Skeletal deformities such as kyphoscoliosis and pes cavus may develop. Electromyography generally shows only nonspecific myopathic changes. The serum muscle enzymes may be normal or only mildly elevated. Both autosomal-dominant and autosomal-recessive patterns of inheritance have been described, in addition to apparently sporadic cases. Histologic studies on muscle specimens from these patients disclose centrally located nuclei in a large but variable number of the myofibers. These can be seen equally as well in both paraffin-embedded and frozen sections (Figs. 8–12 and 8–13). Often the central nuclei appear to be surrounded by small vacuoles that may contain glycogen or lipofuscin. In some patients, the internal nuclei are found in fibers of both types, while in others they are confined to the type I myofibers.[40] Fiber typing also demonstrates predominance of type I myofibers in some of the patients (Fig. 8–14). Furthermore, the type I myofibers are often smaller than the remaining type II myofibers. Several stains, including H&E, trichrome, and especially the NADH–TR reaction, disclose radial striations in cross-sections of the myofibers. These are most prominent in myofibers that are sectioned between internal nuclei (Fig. 8–15). Headington et al.[41] have suggested that this appearance is due to the presence of abnormally small myofibrils in the core of the myofiber around and between successive central nuclei (Fig. 8–16). In addition to the internal nuclei, electron microscopy will often disclose abundant glycogen granules, mitochondria, and membranes derived from the sarcoplasmic reticulum and T-tubules within the central portion of the myofiber.

Other cases of myotubular myopathy do not become clinically evident until adulthood.[36,41,43,44] Most of these patients have mild to moderate weakness affecting the lower limbs more than the upper limbs. In one family, the disease presented as a facioperoneal syndrome.[45] Some, but not all, of the adult patients have had impairment of extraocular mobility. The adult form of the disease usually appears to be transmitted as an autosomal-dominant trait. Muscle spec-

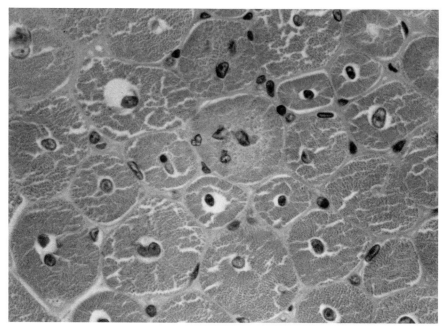

Figure 8-12. Centronuclear myopathy in a 31-year-old woman with moderate weakness documented since adolescence. The patient had an affected daughter and a normal son. Internal, centrally located nuclei are present in a large proportion of the myofibers. The perinuclear vacuoles are, in part, an artifact of paraffin embedment. H&E, ×410.

imens from these patients show an increased number of central nuclei and occasionally contain additional internal nuclei that are not centrally located. The central nuclei may be found in both type I and type II myofibers. In some patients, the type I myofibers are far more numerous and smaller than the type II myofibers, which may be hypertrophied.

The pathogenesis of this condition remains unclear. The original hypothesis of myofiber maturation arrested at the myotubular stage, has been vigorously disputed by many authors but is still supported by others.[44,45] Abnormalities of innervation have been suggested but extrajunctional acetylcholine receptor has not been demonstrated[7,44] and no abnormalities of the spinal cord have been demonstrated at the time of autopsy.[39]

CONGENITAL FIBER-TYPE DISPROPORTION

Congenital fiber-type disproportion was delineated as a distinct congenital myopathy in 1973 by Brooke.[46] The characteristic morphologic features had been noted in the course of an earlier histochemical survey of childhood muscle

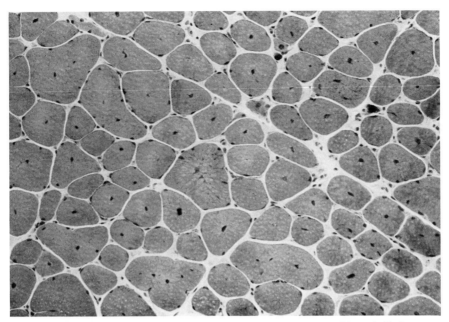

Figure 8–13. Centronuclear myopathy in a 25-year-old man with a similarly affected brother. Both patients had moderate weakness since infancy and were unable to participate in sports. Note the large numbers of central nuclei and variation in myofiber sizes. Trichrome, ×200.

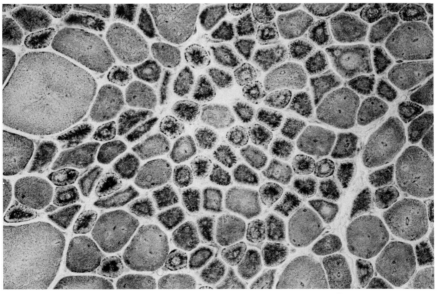

Figure 8–14. Centronuclear myopathy in a 24-year-old man, brother of patient shown in Figure 8–13. Fiber-typing stains show a predominance of type I myofibers. NADH–TR, ×200.

191

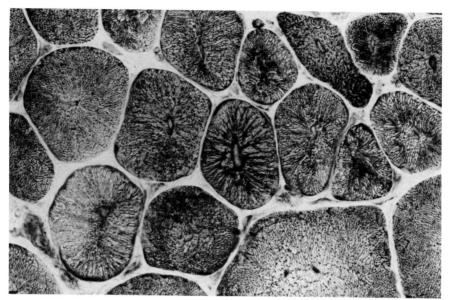

Figure 8-15. Abnormalities in the arrangement of the intermyofibrillar network often impart an appearance of radial striations to cross-sections of the myofibers. NADH–TR, ×500.

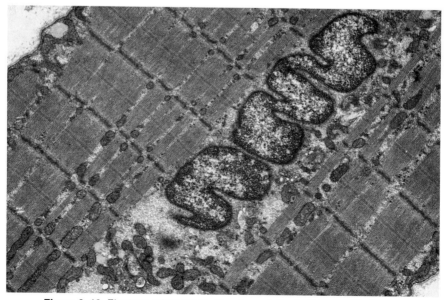

Figure 8-16. Electron micrograph showing relatively thin myofibrils surrounding the centrally located nuclei. ×14,000.

biopsy specimens by Brooke and Engel.[47] A number of cases have been reported subsequently, confirming and expanding the original observations.[48-51] Children affected with this disorder are hypotonic, weak, and have delayed motor development. The patients are often short and have a long thin face with a high arched palate. Congenitally dislocated hips and contractures may be evident in infancy. Proximal weakness is most pronounced during the first 2 years of life. Kyphoscoliosis and spinal rigidity may become apparent as the children get older. Although the condition was originally considered relatively benign, more recent publications have documented residual defects in virtually all of the patients. Some of the cases are familial and an autosomal-dominant pattern of inheritance has been suggested.[49] Argov et al.[51] have suggested that this disease as well as certain other disorders with fiber-type disproportion are the result of altered innervation and impaired maturation of type I or type II motor units.

Morphologically, congenital fiber-type disproportion is characterized by a discrepancy in the size of otherwise normal type I and type II myofibers (Fig. 8-17). Characteristically, the type I myofibers are smaller than the type II my-

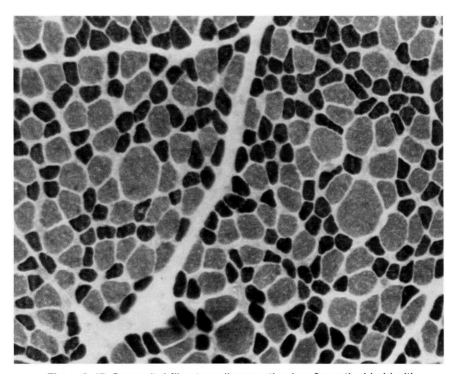

Figure 8-17. Congenital fiber-type disproportion in a 9-month-old girl with weakness and hypotonia. The type I myofibers are significantly smaller than the type II myofibers. ATPase following preincubation at pH 4.3, ×410.

ofibers by 12 percent or more. This is most dramatically shown in histograms that display two distinct peaks. Dubowitz has further suggested that the diagnosis should be made only when the type II myofibers are of normal size or are hypertrophied.[12] In addition to the abnormalities in fiber size, there is often type I myofiber predominance. These features are best demonstrated in sections stained with the ATPase reactions.

Although this pattern of myofiber size discrepancy is typical of congenital fiber-type disproportion, it is not unique to this disorder. Eisler and Wilson[52] have reported a family in which two members had slowly progressive proximal muscle weakness beginning at ages 2 and 6 years. These two symptomatic teenagers and other asymptomatic family members had type I myofiber predominance, small type I myofibers, and minimally enlarged type II myofibers. None of these individuals had congenital hypotonia. Although morphologically similar, these authors considered this disorder different than the congenital fiber-type disproportion described by Brooke. Similar abnormalities of myofiber size also have been reported in children with a wide variety of other neuromuscular diseases including infantile facioscapulohumeral dystrophy,[1] Pompe's disease,[53] the fetal alcohol syndrome,[53] and Krabbe's disease.[53,54]

REDUCING BODY MYOPATHY

This morphologically distinctive disorder was originally described as a congenital myopathy in 1972 by Brooke and Neville.[55] Their two patients were hypotonic female infants who experienced progressive generalized weakness and eventually died at the ages of 9 months and 2½ years, respectively. Subsequently, similar morphologic features have been encountered in older patients with varied clinical manifestations. These have included a scapuloperoneal syndrome,[56] a case clinically resembling an inflammatory myopathy,[57] and cases of benign, nonprogressive myopathy.[58,59]

Muscle specimens from these patients have shown variation in myofiber size, occasional degenerating myofibers, and type I myofiber predominance. The morphologically distinctive feature, the so-called reducing bodies, are round to oval structures measuring 10 to 70 μm in maximal diameter. They are found in a variable proportion of the myofibers, generally located at the periphery of the fibers often near myofiber nuclei. They stain bright red with H&E and reddish–purple with the modified trichrome reaction. They are further characterized histochemically by staining for glycogen, nucleic acids, and sulfhydryl groups. The latter component is best demonstrated by the menadione–nitroblue tetrazolium technique.[55] The bodies are outlined but unstained by the ATPase reactions.

Ultrastructurally, the reducing bodies appear as unbounded masses of osmiophilic granular and fibrillar material in which there are irregular lacunae. The granules range from 15 to 20 nm in diameter while the fibrils measure 12 to 18 nm in diameter. The composition of the bodies is unknown although derivations from ribosomes, viral particles, or myofibrillar components have been suggested.[55,58]

FINGERPRINT BODY MYOPATHY

This nonprogressive or slowly progressive congenital myopathy was first delineated in 1972 by Engel et al.[60] Only a small number of additional cases have been reported subsequently.[61,62] The patients display weakness and hypotonia of limb and axial muscles while the cranial muscles tend to be unaffected. Motor development is delayed. Some of the patients also have been mentally retarded.

Light microscopy of muscle specimens from these individuals discloses myofiber atrophy and type I myofiber predominance. In addition to these relatively nonspecific features, there are numerous small inclusion bodies that are characteristic of this disorder. These bodies are seen as indistinct ovoids, 1 to 10 μm in maximal diameter, that stain reddish with H&E and green with the modified trichrome procedure. They are more clearly seen when the sections are examined by phase microscopy. The inclusion bodies are found predominantly in type I myofibers.

Electron microscopy has shown the inclusions to be composed of roughly parallel osmiophilic lamellae that are arranged in complex patterns resembling fingerprints. The individual lamellae have a serrated appearance. The composition of these structures is unknown. It has been suggested that they may be derived from myofibrillar proteins[60] or degenerating mitochondria.[62]

Although these structures are the characteristic morphologic feature of fingerprint body myopathy, ultrastructurally identical inclusions have been found in other diseases, including myotonic dystrophy, oculopharyngeal dystrophy, and inflammatory myopathy.[62]

CYTOPLASMIC BODY MYOPATHY

Cytoplasmic bodies are found as a nonspecific alteration in a wide variety of diverse disorders. These include inflammatory myopathies, periodic paralyses, myotonic dystrophy, denervation, and various toxic and metabolic myopathies. They are also the morphologic hallmark of a presumably congenital neuromyopathy.[63–65] To date, only a small number of cases have been reported. The condition may be sporadic or familial with onset at any age between the neonatal period and early adulthood. The disease is manifested by proximal or generalized weakness and may be static or progressive leading to respiratory complications. Some of the patients have also had a cardiomyopathy.

Muscle specimens from these patients have shown increased variation in myofiber size and type I myofiber predominance. Numerous cytoplasmic bodies, the single morphologic feature common among these patients, were found predominantly in type I myofibers. This is in contrast to the more frequent occurrence of cytoplasmic bodies in type II myofibers when they are associated with other disorders.

By light microscopy, cytoplasmic bodies are seen most clearly with the modified trichrome procedure. With this technique, they appear as small, dense red masses surrounded by a pale–green halo (see Fig. 3–5). They can also be seen, but less clearly, with H&E in which case they stain red and are surrounded by a pink halo. The bodies and the surrounding halos are unstained by the NADH–TR and ATPase techniques.

By electron microscopy, cytoplasmic bodies appear to consist of a core of osmiophilic, finely granular material surrounded by a corona of thin filaments (see Fig. 3–6). In some instances, they appear to arise at the level of the Z-disc. Derivations from Z-discs[66] and from myofilaments[65] have been suggested.

SPHEROID BODY MYOPATHY

Another disorder that may be closely related to cytoplasmic body myopathy is so-called "spheroid body myopathy." This slowly progressive, autosomal-dominant disease was delineated by Goebel et al. in 1978.[67] The spheroid bodies that morphologically characterize the disease are rounded structures that measure 2 to 15 μm in diameter. They often occur in large aggregates and are found predominantly in type I myofibers. They stain green by the modified trichrome technique but remain unstained by most other procedures. Ultrastructurally, they appear as compact, swirled masses of fine filaments that measure 12 to 15 nm in diameter. In contrast to cytoplasmic bodies, they lack a central core of granular osmiophilic material.

CONGENITAL HYPOTONIA AND TYPE I MYOFIBER PREDOMINANCE

In 1957, Walton[68] had used the term "benign congenital hypotonia" to describe hypotonic infants with a relatively benign course who did not fit into other recognized disease categories. Although all these infants had delayed motor development, many eventually recovered fully. Others were left with mild to moderate disabilities including kyphoscoliosis. Morphologic studies of paraffin-embedded muscle specimens from these patients failed to show any abnormalities. Similar cases, included in the comprehensive histochemical survey of children's muscle biopsies by Brooke and Engel,[47] were observed to have type I myofiber predominance without atrophy or other morphologic abnormalities.

More recently, Brooke[69] restricted the term "benign congenital hypotonia" to infants with normal muscle morphology and hypotonia as their only clinical manifestation. These children had a uniformly favorable prognosis. By contrast, muscle specimens from other hypotonic children displayed type I my-

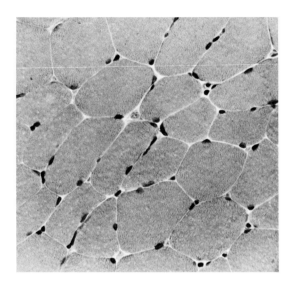

Figure 8-18. Type I myofiber predominance in a 12-year-old boy with scoliosis. The muscle fibers show no structural abnormalities. H&E, ×410.

ofiber predominance. Some of these children displayed additional clinical manifestations. These included decreased tendon reflexes, mild skeletal anomalies, and mild weakness that persisted into adult life. Other authors also have reported older children and adults with congenital nonprogressive neuromuscular disease with a very high proportion of type I myofibers as the only morphologic abnormality.[70,71] The occurrence in siblings has suggested that the disease is familial. We have studied two patients, a child with scoliosis and an adult with a lifelong, nonprogressive myopathy in whom type I predominance was the only recognized abnormality (Figs. 8–18 and 8–19). These cases

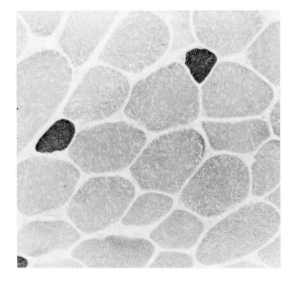

Figure 8-19. Type I myofiber predominance, same patient as in Figure 8–18. With the fiber-typing stains, marked type I myofiber predominance is evident. ATPase, ×410.

must be distinguished carefully from neurogenic diseases with type I predominance.

PRADER–WILLI SYNDROME

The Prader–Willi syndrome is another cause of congential hypotonia that can masquerade as primary neuromuscular disease. As young infants, these patients are often small and have feeding difficulties. The diagnosis may not be evident until abnormal weight gain begins about the time when the children begin to walk. Muscle biopsies from these patients are generally reported to show no significant morphologic abnormalities.

References

1. Brooke MH, Carroll JE, Ringel SP: Congenital hypotonia revisited. Muscle Nerve 2:84–100, 1979.
2. Shy GM, Magee KR: A new congenital non-progressive myopathy. Brain 76:610–621, 1956.
3. Telerman-Toppet N, Gerard JM, Coers C: Central core disease: A study of clinically unaffected muscle. J Neurol Sci 19:207–223, 1973.
4. Frank JP, Harati Y, Butler IJ, et al.: Central core disease and malignant hyperthermia syndrome. Ann Neurol 7:11–17, 1980.
5. Neville HE, Brooke MH: Central core fibers: Structured and unstructured. In Kakulas BA (ed): Basic Research in Myology. Amsterdam, Excerpta Medica, 1973, pp 497–511.
6. Afifi AK, Smith JW, Zellweger H: Congenital non-progressive myopathy. Central core disease and nemaline myopathy in one family. Neurology 15:371–381, 1965.
7. Ringel SP, Bender AN, Engel WK: Extrajunctional acetylcholine receptors. Alterations in human and experimental neuromuscular diseases. Arch Neurol 33:751–758, 1976.
8. Karpati G, Carpenter S, Eisen AA: Experimental core-like lesions and nemaline rods. A correlative morphological and physiological study. Arch Neurol 27:237–251, 1972.
9. Carpenter S, Karpati G: Pathology of Skeletal Muscle. New York, Churchill Livingstone, 1984, pp 434–441.
10. Engel AG, Gomez MR, Groover RV: Multicore disease. A recently recognized congenital myopathy associated with multifocal degeneration of muscle fibers. Mayo Clin Proc 46:666–681, 1971.
11. Heffner R, Cohen M, Duffner P, Daigler G: Multicore disease in twins. J Neurol Neurosurg Psychiatry 39:602–606, 1976.
12. Dubowitz V: Muscle Disorders in Childhood. London, Saunders, 1978, pp, 70–107.
13. Bonnette H, Roelofs R, Olson WH: Multicore disease: Report of a case with onset in middle age. Neurology 24:1039-1044, 1974.
14. Conen PE, Murphy EG, Donohue WL: Light and electron microscopic studies of "myogranules" in a child with hypotonia and muscle weakness. Can Med Assoc J 89:983–986, 1963.
15. Shy GM, Engel WK, Somers JE, Wanko T: Nemaline myopathy. A new congenital myopathy. Brain 86:793–810, 1963.

16. Neustein HB: Nemaline myopathy. A family study with three autopsied cases. Arch Pathol 96:192–195, 1973.

17. Gillies C, Raye J, Vasan U, et al.: Nemaline (rod) myopathy. A possible cause of rapidly fatal infantile hypotonia. Arch Pathol Lab Med 103:1–5, 1979.

18. Norton P, Ellison P, Sulaiman AR, Harb J: Nemaline myopathy in the neonate. Neurology 33:351–356, 1983.

19. Heffernan LP, Rewcastle NB, Humphrey JG: The spectrum of rod myopathy. Arch Neurol 18:529–542, 1986.

20. Engel WK, Oberc MA: Abundant nuclear rods in adult-onset rod disease. J Neuropathol Exp Neurol 34:119–132, 1975.

21. Kinoshita M, Satoyoshi E: Type I fiber atrophy and nemaline bodies. Arch Neurol 31:423–425, 1974.

22. Brownell AKW, Gilbert JJ, Shaw DT, et al.: Adult onset nemaline myopathy. Neurology 28:1306–1309, 1978.

23. Greenwood SM, Viozzi FJ: Nemaline myopathy. Arch Pathol Lab Med 102:196–200, 1978.

24. Danon MJ, Giometti CS, Manaligod JR, et al.: Adult-onset nemaline rods in a patient treated for suspected dermatomyositis. Study with two-dimensional electrophoresis. Arch Neurol 38:761–766, 1981.

25. Jenis EH, Lindquist RR, Lister RC: New congenital myopathy with crystalline intranuclear inclusions. Arch Neurol 20:281–287, 1969.

26. Meier C, Voellmy W, Gertsch M, et al.: Nemaline myopathy appearing in adults as cardiomyopathy. A clinicopathologic study. Arch Neurol 41:443–445, 1984.

27. Kondo K, Yuasa T: Genetics of congenital nemaline myopathy. Muscle Nerve 3:308–315, 1980.

28. Bender AN, Willner JP: Nemaline (rod) myopathy: The need for histochemical evaluation of affected families. Ann Neurol 4:37–42, 1978.

29. Karpati G, Carpenter S, Andermann F: A new concept of childhood nemaline myopathy. Arch Neurol 24:291–304, 1971.

30. Engel AG, Gomez MR: Nemaline (Z-disk) myopathy: Observations on the origin, structure, and solubility properties of the nemaline structures. J Neuropathol Exp Neurol 26:601–619, 1967.

31. Stuhlfauth I, Jennekens FGI, Willemse J, Jockusch BM: Congenital nemaline myopathy. II. Quantitative changes in α-actinin and myosin in skeletal muscle. Muscle Nerve 6:69–74, 1983.

32. Jennekens FGI, Roord JJ, Veldman H, et al: Congenital nemaline myopathy. I. Defective organization of α-actinin is restricted to muscle. Muscle Nerve 6:61–68, 1983.

33. Martinez AJ, Hay S, McNeer KW: Extraocular muscles: Light microscopy and ultrastructural features. Acta Neuropathol 34:237–253, 1976.

34. Spiro AJ, Shy GM, Gonatas NK: Myotubular myopathy—persistence of fetal muscle in an adolescent boy. Arch Neurol 14:1–14, 1966.

35. Sher JH, Rimalovski AB, Athanassiades TJ, Aronson SM: Familial centronuclear myopathy: A clinical and pathological study. Neurology 17:727–742, 1967.

36. Schochet SS Jr, Zellweger H, Ionasescu V, McCormick WF: Centronuclear myopathy: Disease entity or a syndrome? Light and electron-microscopy study of two cases and review of the literature. J Neurol Sci 16:215–228, 1972.

37. van Wijngaarden GK, Fleury P, Bethlem J, Meijer AEFH: Familial "myotubular" myopathy. Neurology 19:901–908, 1969.

38. Barth PG, van Wijngaarden GK, Bethlem J: X-linked myotubular myopathy with fatal neonatal asphyxia. Neurology 25:531–536, 1975.

39. Engel WK, Gold GN, Karpati G: Type I fiber hypotrophy and central nuclei. A rare congenital muscle abnormality with a possible experimental model. Arch Neurol 18:435–444, 1968.

40. Karpati G, Carpenter S, Nelson RF: Type I muscle fiber atrophy and central nuclei. A rare familial neuromuscular disease. J Neurol Sci 10:489–500, 1970.

41. Headington JT, McNamara JO, Brownell AK: Centronuclear myopathy: Histochemistry and electron microscopy. Report of two cases. Arch Pathol 99:16-24, 1975.

42. Serratrice G, Pellissier JF, Faugere MC, Gastaut JL: Centronuclear myopathy: Possible central nervous system origin. Muscle Nerve 1:62–69, 1978.

43. McLeod JG, Baker WC, Lethlean AK, Shorey CD: Centronuclear myopathy with autosomal dominant inheritance. J Neurol Sci 15:375–387, 1972.

44. Bergen BJ, Carry MP, Wilson WB, et al.: Centronuclear myopathy: Extraocular and limb–muscle findings in an adult. Muscle Nerve 3:165–171, 1980.

45. Edstrom L, Wroblewski R, Mair WGP: Genuine myotubular myopathy. Muscle Nerve 5:604–613, 1982.

46. Brooke MH: Congenital fiber type disproportion. In Kakulas BA (ed): Clinical Studies in Myology, Part 2. Amsterdam, Excerpta Medica, 1973, pp 147–159.

47. Brooke MH, Engel WK: The histographic analysis of human muscle biopsies with regard to fiber types. 4. Children's biopsies. Neurology 19:591–605, 1969.

48. Lendard HG, Goebel HH: Congenital fibre type disproportion. Neuropaediatrie 6:220–231, 1975.

49. Curless RG, Nelson MB: Congenital fiber type disproportion in identical twins. Ann Neurol 2:455–459, 1977.

50. Clancy RR, Kelts KA, Dehlert JW: Clinical variability in congenital fiber type disproportion. J Neurol Sci 46:257–266, 1980.

51. Argov Z, Gardner-Medwin D, Johnson MA, Mastaglia FL: Patterns of muscle fiber-type disproportion in hypotonic infants. Arch Neurol 41:53–57, 1984.

52. Eisler T, Wilson JH: Muscle fiber-type disproportion. Report of a family with symptomatic and asymptomatic members. Arch Neurol 35:823–826, 1978.

53. Martin JJ, Clara R, Ceuterick C, Joris C: Is congenital fiber type disproportion a true myopathy? Acta Neurol Belg 76:335–344, 1976.

54. Dehkharghani F, Sarnat HB, Brewster MA, Roth SI: Congenital muscle fiber-type disproportion in Krabbe's leukodystrophy. Arch Neurol 38:585–587, 1981.

55. Brooke MH, Neville HE: Reducing body myopathy. Neurology 22:829–840, 1972.

56. Sahgal V, Sahgal S: A new congenital myopathy: A morphological, cytochemical and histochemical study. Acta Neuropathol 37:225–230, 1977.

57. Dubowitz V: Muscle Disorders in Childhood. London, Saunders, 1978, pp 219–221.

58. Tome FMS, Fardeau M: Congenital myopathy with "reducing bodies" in muscle fibres. Acta Neuropathol 31:207–217, 1975.

59. Oh SJ, Meyers GJ, Wilson ER Jr, Alexander CB: A benign form of reducing body myopathy. Muscle Nerve 6:278–282, 1983.

60. Engel AG, Angelini C, Gomez MR: Fingerprint body myopathy. A newly recognized congenital muscle disease. Mayo Clin Proc 47:377–388, 1972.

61. Fardeau M, Tome FMS, Derambure S: Familial fingerprint body myopathy. Arch Neurol 33:724–725, 1976.

62. Curless RG, Payne CM, Brinner FM: Fingerprint body myopathy. A report of twins. Dev Med Child Neurol 20:793–798, 1978.

63. Jerusalem F, Ludin H, Bischoff A, Hartmann G: Cytoplasmic body neuromyopathy presenting as respiratory failure and weight loss. J Neurol Sci 41:1-9, 1979.

64. Goebel HH, Schloon H, Lenard HG: Congenital myopathy with cytoplasmic bodies. Neuropediatrics 12:166–180, 1981.
65. Wolburg H, Schlote W, Langohr HD, et al.: Slowly progressive congenital myopathy with cytoplasmic bodies—report of two cases and a review of the literature. Clin Neuropathol 1:55–66, 1982.
66. MacDonald RD, Engel AG: The cytoplasmic body: Another structural anomaly of the Z-disc. Acta Neuropathol 14:99–107, 1969.
67. Goebel HH, Muller J, Gillen HW, Merritt AD: Autosomal dominant "spheroid body myopathy." Muscle Nerve 1:14–26, 1978.
68. Walton JN: The limp child. J Neurol Neurosurg Psychiatry 20:144–154, 1957.
69. Brooke MH: A Clinician's View of Neuromuscular Diseases. Baltimore, Williams & Wilkins, 1977, pp 200–202.
70. Oh SJ, Danon MJ: Nonprogressive congenital neuromuscular disease with uniform type I fiber. Arch Neurol 40:147–150, 1983.
71. Vallat JM, Lagueny A, Luchmaya K, et al.: Nonprogressive congenital neuromuscular disease with uniform type I fiber. Arch Neurol 40:828–829, 1983.

chapter 9

Peripheral Nerves

Peripheral neuropathies are commonly encountered disorders that often prove to be diagnostic conundrums. Although neuropathies may be isolated disorders, they are more often a manifestation of an underlying systemic disease. Unfortunately, the etiology of many clinically apparent neuropathies has not been established with certainty. Despite the major advances that have come from investigative techniques employed by various research groups, routine histopathologic examinations of peripheral nerve specimens often yield disappointingly limited information. Several factors contribute to this problem:

1. Only a few peripheral nerves lend themselves to biopsy and these are predominantly sensory nerves.
2. Peripheral nerves are not adequately sampled during routine autopsies.
3. Peripheral nerves exhibit a limited spectrum of morphologic alterations which are often similar regardless of the etiology of the neuropathy.
4. Multiple specialized techniques must be employed in order to examine a peripheral nerve specimen comprehensively.
5. Detailed genetic, clinical, electrophysiologic, and laboratory data must be obtained for correlation with the morphologic findings.

PERIPHERAL NERVE BIOPSIES

Peripheral nerve biopsies should be performed only after careful consideration of their potential contribution to patient management since the procedure itself will invariably result in at least some degree of a neurologic deficit. Most authors[1-3] agree that nerve biopsies are most helpful in the evaluation of diseases that produce multiple mononeuropathies. Typical examples would include the various forms of vasculitis and Hansen's disease. Nerve biopsies may be useful in the evaluation of certain genetically determined metabolic diseases such as Krabbe's disease, metachromatic leukodystrophy, adrenoleukodystrophy, Fabry's disease, and the neuronal ceroid lipofuscinoses. Although biochemical procedures are now available for the diagnosis of several of these diseases, the serious implications of the diagnosis justify morphologic confirmation. In the case of the neuronal ceroid lipofuscinoses, reliable biochemical procedures are not yet available and a morphologic diagnosis can often be established readily from a nerve biopsy specimen. Evaluation of certain demyelinating disorders, especially chronic forms with hypertrophied nerves, often can be facilitated by morphologic examination of biopsy specimens. Biopsies are generally less informative when performed on patients with symmetrical distal polyneuropathies due to systemic metabolic diseases or intoxications. These specimens generally show an admixture of nonspecific changes reflecting both axonal degeneration and secondary segmental demyelination. Unfortunately, a large proportion of nerve biopsy specimens fall into this last category. Noteworthy exceptions to this generalization are amyloidosis and a few toxic and metabolic disorders that give rise to morphologically distinctive giant axonal neuropathies.

BIOPSY PROCEDURES

The sural nerve is the most readily accessible and commonly biopsied peripheral nerve. Since it is a sensory nerve except for a small number of unmyelinated autonomic fibers, the neurologic deficit from the biopsy procedure itself will be limited to an area of anesthesia on the lateral aspect of the foot. Some authors advocate removal of a nerve fascicle rather than the whole nerve in order to minimize the resulting neurologic deficit. However, the surgical procedure is more difficult and often yields a specimen with numerous traumatic artifacts. Furthermore, some authors doubt that there is any significant difference in the degree of long-term sensory loss.[4] In either case, the specimen should be at least 2 to 3 cm in length in order to provide sufficient tissue for a variety of histopathologic techniques. Upon removal, the biopsy specimen should be wrapped in saline-moistened gauze and taken promptly to the histology laboratory for processing.

Parenthetically, it should be mentioned that a good muscle biopsy specimen, obtained from the motor end point, will often contain small branches of motor nerves (Fig. 9–1). These nerve twigs should not be overlooked in the evaluation of patients with peripheral neuropathies. They are the most readily available source of motor nerves that can be obtained by biopsy. The intramuscular nerve twigs may show increased endoneurial fibrosis in patients with denervating diseases such as the spinal muscular atrophies and various axonal neuropathies.[5] Occasionally other, more specific morphologic features may be encountered.

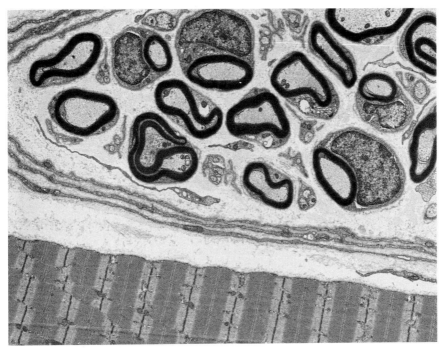

Figure 9-1. Electron micrograph of an intramuscular nerve twig within a muscle biopsy specimen. This potentially valuable source of nerve specimens should not be overlooked when evaluating neuromuscular diseases. ×6000.

AUTOPSY PROCEDURES

Because of the real or presumed restrictions of the usual routine autopsy permission, much of the peripheral nervous system is regarded as inaccessible by the prosector. Nevertheless, certain structures may be sampled with ease without additional incisions. These include spinal nerve roots, the cauda equina, dorsal root ganglia, and portions of the brachial and lumbar plexi. Sural nerves can be obtained with a minimum of extra dissection. In patients with known peripheral neuropathies, potentially valuable information could be obtained by sampling peripheral nerves at multiple levels. Special permission can be requested for these more extensive examinations.

SPECIMEN PREPARATION

In the histopathology laboratory, the nerve specimens should be divided into several appropriate portions for further processing. Conventional paraffin-embedded sections, epoxy-embedded sections, and individual teased nerve fibers should be prepared from every nerve biopsy specimen. When indicated, electron microscopy can also be performed on the epoxy-embedded tissue. If sufficient tissue is available, frozen sections may be useful. The specimen intended for paraffin embedment should be placed on a piece of thin cardboard or on a frosted glass slide in order to keep it oriented properly during formalin fixation. Prior to the actual paraffin embedment, a small portion should be cut off and oriented so that both transverse and longitudinal sections can be obtained. The specimen should not be cut up excessively. The minimal routine battery of stains should include H&E, trichrome, and Congo Red procedures. A myelin sheath stain such as luxol fast blue and an axon stain such as the Bodian procedure also may be useful. Because of nonspecific staining of endoneurial collagen, the latter stains are often more difficult to interpret when performed on peripheral nerves than on specimens from the central nervous system. The Gomori trichrome stain, with its red myelin and green connective tissue (Fig. 9-2), often displays the myelin sheaths of peripheral nerves better than the traditional myelin stains. Many luxol-fast blue preparations stain peripheral nerve myelin greener than the myelin in the central nervous system. This has been attributed to differences in the cerebroside content. Congo Red

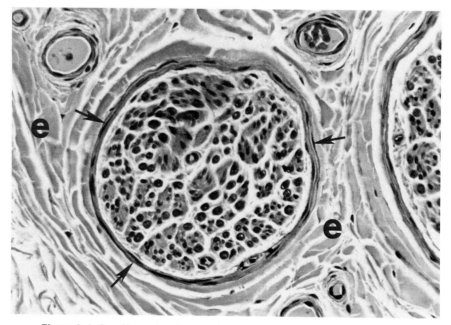

Figure 9-2. Paraffin-embedded sural nerve biopsy specimen. Epineurial connective tissue (e) surrounds the nerve and extends between the nerve fascicles. The individual nerve fascicles are bounded by the perineurium (arrows). The myelin sheaths are stained bright red (dark in the photograph) in contrast to the green endoneurium, perineurium, and epineurium. Trichrome, ×410.

preparations must be thoroughly differentiated in order to remove excess stain bound nonspecifically to the collagen. Furthermore, the characteristic yellow–green birefringence colors must be demonstrated by examination with polarized light before any staining is accepted as indicating the presence of amyloid. Equivocal cases can be resolved best by electron microscopy.

Tissue for the epoxy-embedded sections and the individual teased nerve fiber preparations should be fixed initially in glutaraldehyde. After adequate fixation, one can longitudinally section this segment of the nerve biopsy specimen and obtain portions for the individual teased nerve fiber preparations and for the epoxy-embedded blocks. We prepare these blocks by the same techniques that we employ for muscle. For light microscopy, sections 1 to 2 μm in thickness are stained with toluidine blue or paraphenylenediamine. A relatively large number of blocks, i.e., more than 20, should be prepared in order to minimize sampling errors and facilitate examination of representative longitudinal and cross-sections (Fig. 9–3). The latter sections are especially useful for evaluating changes in the population of nerve fibers, e.g., selective loss of small or large nerve fibers. When indicated, the distribution of fiber sizes can be quantitated and the data can be portrayed graphically with histograms. When needed, the same epoxy-embedded blocks can be sectioned further for electron

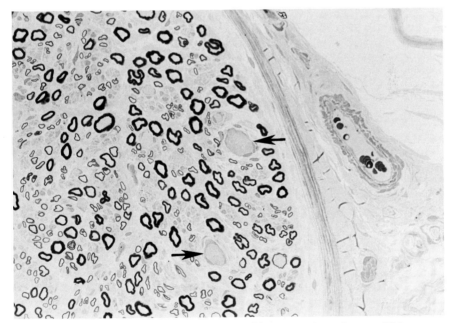

Figure 9–3. Epoxy-embedded sural nerve biopsy specimen from a child with giant axonal neuropathy. These sections are especially useful for evaluating the variation in size of the myelinated nerve fibers. Two of the so-called giant axonal enlargements can be seen *(arrows)*. Paraphenylenediamine, ×500.

microscopy. This is the most accurate way to evaluate the small unmyelinated nerve fibers, to detect lysosomal storage deposits in Schwann cells and axons, to confirm the presence of amyloid and so forth.

Often the most informative of histopathologic techniques for evaluation of peripheral nerves is the preparation of individual teased nerve fibers (Fig. 9–4). These are relatively tedious and time-consuming to prepare but should be performed on every specimen. Dyck et al.[3] have developed a detailed classification and grading system for the full spectrum of abnormalities that may be seen in these preparations. However, even when performed and examined by less-experienced individuals, otherwise subtle changes of segmental demyelination, remyelination, and axonal degeneration become conspicuous.

For these preparations, a segment of nerve at least 1 cm long is fixed initially in cacodylate-buffered, 4 percent glutaraldehyde and then postfixed in a cacodylate-buffered, 1 percent osmium tetroxide solution. As indicated previously, we often longitudinally split the specimen so that it can also be used for epoxy embedment. The nerve is then soaked overnight in 50 percent glycerol followed by another 12 to 24 hours in pure glycerol. With the investigator working with pointed forceps under a dissecting microscope, the epineurium and perineurium are removed. The fascicles of nerve fibers are then separated until individual nerve fibers or small groups of two to three nerve fibers can be teased from the fascicle. Several different fascicles should be sampled. The individual teased nerve fibers can be pulled onto another slide, accompanied by a minimum of glycerol. We generally prepare four slides, each containing

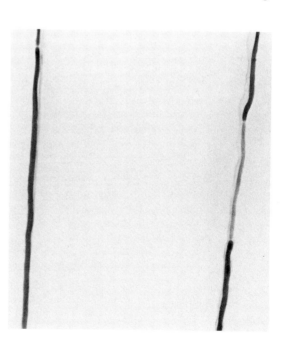

Figure 9-4. Teased nerve fiber preparation from a 47-year-old man with a chronic demyelinating neuropathy. Note the short, thinly myelinated internode on the fiber to the right. × 175.

about 25 teased nerve fibers. We coverslip two slides with regular mounting medium and two with glycerol. The latter preparations are not permanent but are especially useful if the teased nerve fibers are to be photographed. Occasionally, we have found it useful to accentuate the staining of the nerve fibers by treating them with a paraphenylenediamine solution. In general, we have found it much more difficult to prepare teased nerve fibers from autopsy specimens than from biopsy specimens.

If sufficient tissue is available, frozen sections may be useful. We generally prepare both cross-sections and longitudinal sections by standing a very short transverse segment along side of a short longitudinal segment. These are rapidly frozen with liquid nitrogen. The sections are stained by H&E, modified trichrome, PAS, and nonspecific esterase using the same techniques as employed with muscle specimens. In general, sections stained by the modified trichrome procedure prove to be the most useful. The myelin sheaths stain red to orange in contrast to the green connective tissue. The nonspecific esterase reaction will accentuate areas of phagocytic activity regardless of the cause. Rarely, we employ the crystal violet stain on frozen sections to detect amyloid. Generally, we find the Congo Red stain on paraffin-embedded sections more satisfactory. The Hirsch–Peiffer stain, acidified cresyl violet, can be used on the frozen sections when the possibility of metachromatic leukodystrophy is being investigated.

NORMAL PERIPHERAL NERVES AND THEIR ENSHEATHMENTS

The connective tissue sheath that surrounds the exterior of a multifascicular peripheral nerve and extends between the individual fascicles is designated as the *epineurium* (Fig. 9–2). Arterioles, veins, and lymphatics may be found within the fibroadipose tissue comprising this layer. In addition to harboring nutrient blood vessels, this layer of connective tissue contributes to the mechanical strength of the peripheral nerves. Each individual fascicle of a multifascicular nerve is surrounded by the perineurium (Figs. 9–2 and 9–5). This sheath is composed of concentric lamellae of specialized Schwann cells alternating with layers of longitudinally oriented collagen fibers. Within each of the laminae, the Schwann cells are interdigitated and connected to one another by tight junctions. These cells contain numerous pinocytotic vesicles and both surfaces of the Schwann cell lamellae are covered by prominent basement membranes (Fig. 9–5). The perineurium is semipermeable and functions as one component of a blood–nerve barrier.

The term *endoneurium* is variously employed to designate all components of the nerve, including the nerve fibers, bounded by perineurium, or as used, here, the intrafascicular connective tissues. The majority of the nuclei seen within the endoneurium are Schwann cell nuclei. The remainder belong to

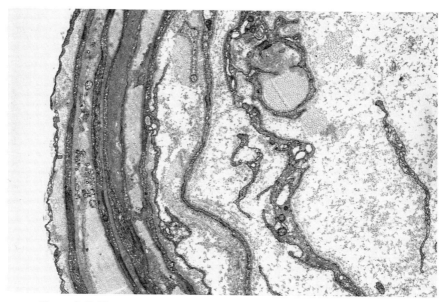

Figure 9-5. Electron micrograph of the perineurium. This sheath is composed of concentric lamellae of Schwann cell processes and layers of longitudinally oriented collagen fibrils. ×9000.

fibroblasts and mast cells. The fibroblast nuclei are generally more varied in shape than the Schwann cell nuclei and are accompanied by irregular elongated cytoplasmic processes. Ultrastructurally, the fibroblasts are readily distinguished by the lack of a prominent basement membrane that regularly surrounds the Schwann cells. Although relatively inconspicuous, mast cells are frequently encountered within peripheral nerves both within the endoneurium and in the epineurium. They are relatively inconspicuous in sections stained by the usual techniques but can be demonstrated vividly in sections stained with toluidine blue. This procedure stains the mast cell granules metachromatically, i.e., reddish–purple. The role of mast cells in the normal nerve and in various pathologic processes where they appear more numerous, is unclear. Histamine contained within their granules may influence the permeability of endoneurial blood vessels and thereby affect endoneurial pressure. Mast cells often appear to be especially numerous in association with peripheral nerve tumors.

The blood vessels within the endoneurium are semipermeable and comprise the second component of the blood–nerve barrier. This permeability barrier is at least in part due to the tight junctions between the endothelial cells within the vessels. In recent years, there have been extensive investigations into the role of altered endoneurial permeability and role of increased endo-neurial pressure in the development of various peripheral neuropathies.[6,7]

RENAUT CORPUSCLES

Renaut corpuscles are morphologically distinctive structures that may be en-countered in the course of examining peripheral nerve specimens. Bergouignan and Vital[8] found them in about 2 percent of peroneal nerve biopsy specimens. The Renaut corpuscles are fusiform subperineurial masses that bulge into the endoneurium (Fig. 9-6). They are sparsely cellular and appear laminated or whorled in cross-section. They are composed of abundant hyalinized or mucoid material in which there are stellate or flattened fibroblasts with large vesicular nuclei. The mucoid or hyaline matrix stains strongly with alcian blue, reflect-ing the presence of abundant acid mucopolysaccharides. Electron microscopy discloses the presence of numerous fine filaments within an amorphous gran-ular matrix. Although originally described in 1881, they were often ignored or misinterpreted as nerve infarcts or amyloid deposits, as pointed out by Asbury.[9] It has been suggested that they are especially common in segments of periph-eral nerve subjected to compression and trauma. This has received some sup-

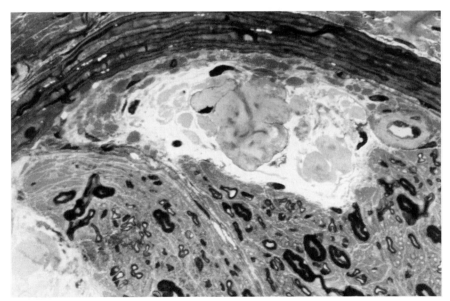

Figure 9-6. Epoxy section showing a subperineurial Renaut corpuscle. These must not be misinterpreted as deposits of amyloid. Toluidine blue, ×800.

port from the experimental studies reported by Ortman et al.[10] They may be encountered somewhat more commonly in patients with peripheral neuropathies but are not a specific feature of any particular disorder.

PERIPHERAL NERVE FIBERS

Most of the peripheral nerves that are routinely examined are composed of a mixture of myelinated and unmyelinated nerve fibers, with the unmyelinated fibers being about four times more numerous than the larger myelinated fibers. The myelinated fibers range from about 2 to 22 μm in diameter and show a bimodal distribution of fiber sizes with peaks at about 4 and 11 μm. The relative proportions of the various-sized myelinated fibers are best assessed from examination of epoxy-embedded sections. The unmyelinated fibers range from about 0.4 to 2.4 μm in diameter and have a unimodal size distribution. Although they can be seen by light microscopy, they are best evaluated by electron microscopy. In general, the larger-diameter myelinated fibers have thicker myelin sheaths and longer internodal lengths. For a given fiber size, the myelin thickness and internodal lengths are relatively constant. The largest nerve fibers have an internode length approaching 2.0 mm in length. These are important features to consider when evaluating teased nerve fiber preparations for evidence of remyelination.

A single Schwann cell is associated with each internode of a myelinated nerve fiber. The nucleus of the Schwann cell is located toward the center of the corresponding internode. The periphery of the Schwann cell cytoplasm is surrounded by a prominent basement membrane that extends, without interruption, across the node of Ranvier onto the Schwann cell of the successive internode. The relations of the axon, myelin sheath, and Schwann cell are seen best in transverse sections (Fig. 9–7). The axon is surrounded by a narrow periaxonal space. This in turn is surrounded by a thin layer of adaxonal Schwann cell cytoplasm. The myelin sheath is composed of spiral lamellae derived from the Schwann cell. The lamellae are demarcated by major and minor dense lines with a radial periodicity of about 15 nm. The major dense lines result from the apposition of inner surfaces of the Schwann cell membranes while the minor dense lines result from the apposition of the outer surfaces of the Schwann cell membranes. Except near the Schwann cell nuclei, and to a lesser extent near the nodes of Ranvier, there is only a thin layer of Schwann cell cytoplasm peripheral to the myelin sheath. The Schwann cell cytoplasm may contain osmiophilic, laminated, and granular rod-shaped bodies (Fig. 9–8). These are the so-called pi-granules of Reich. They measure up to 1 μm in length and may be seen by light microscopy as metachromatic granules in sections that are stained with toluidine blue. They are thought to be lysosomes since they also display acid phosphatase activity. They increase in num-

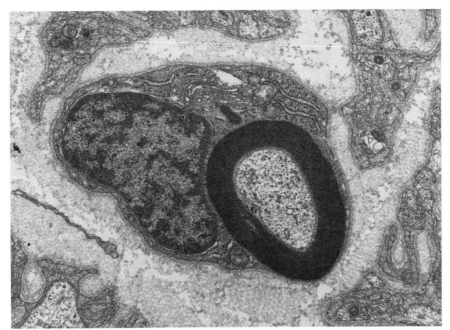

Figure 9-7. Electron micrograph showing a myelinated nerve fiber in transverse section. The section is from near the middle of the internode and shows the nucleus of the Schwann cell from which the myelin sheath is derived. Note the surrounding basement membrane. ×20,000.

ber with aging and are more common in various peripheral neuropathies. Their presence, however, is not indicative of any specific disorder.

Schwann cell cytoplasm is largely excluded from the myelin sheath except in the Schmidt–Lantermann clefts and at the nodes of Ranvier. At the Schmidt–Lantermann clefts, the major dense lines appear to separate and enclose small pockets of Schwann cell cytoplasm. Occasionally, microtubules and desmosomelike structures can be seen within the enclosed cytoplasm. Although the Schmidt–Lantermann clefts appear to be a diagonally oriented series of isolated structures when viewed in longitudinal section, they actually correspond to continuous tongues of Schwann cell cytoplasm that spiral within the myelin sheath. By light microscopy, the Schmidt–Lantermann clefts appear as "arrow-shaped" disruptions in the myelin sheaths. Their number is roughly proportional to the thickness of the myelin sheath and length of the internode. Although their function is unknown, they appear to be selectively vulnerable sites during the breakdown of the myelin sheath under pathologic conditions.

Adjacent to the nodes of Ranvier (Fig. 9–9), the major dense lines again appear to terminate in tongues of Schwann cell cytoplasm. These are arranged so that the more peripheral lamellae terminate in tongues of cytoplasm that

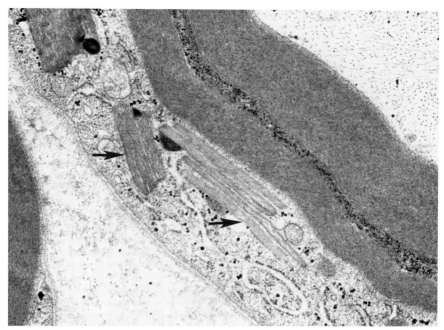

Figure 9-8. Electron micrograph showing laminated rod-shaped pi-granules of Reich within Schwann cell cytoplasm associated with a myelinated axon. Although these structures are nonspecific, they are encountered more commonly in nerve biopsy specimens from patients with chronic neuropathies. ×40,000.

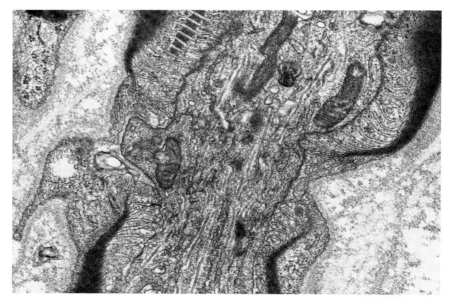

Figure 9-9. Electron micrograph showing a node of Ranvier. The major dense lines of the myelin sheath terminate in tongues of Schwann cell cytoplasm. ×40,000.

extend further toward the midportion of the node. The outer tongue of abaxonal cytoplasm may extend across the node and interdigitate with the tongue of abaxonal cytoplasm from the next internode. Specialized contacts, appearing as a series of osmiophilic densities, may be seen between the tongues of Schwann cell cytoplasm and the underlying axon. The node is also covered by basement membrane that continues without interruption from one internode to the next.

The term "unmyelinated nerve fibers" should be reserved for those small nerve fibers that normally are not invested with a myelin sheath. This is in contrast to demyelinated fibers which are formerly myelinated fibers that have lost their myelin sheath as the result of a pathologic process. The small unmyelinated fibers are more numerous than the larger myelinated fibers but are more difficult to evaluate. Although they can be seen by light microscopy, especially in sections stained by various metallic impregnation techniques, they are displayed to best advantage by electron microscopy. They tend to be unevenly dispersed within the cross-section of a peripheral nerve and are preferentially distributed along with the smaller myelinated fibers. In contrast to the myelinated fibers, several unmyelinated fibers may be invaginated into the cytoplasm of a single Schwann cell (Fig. 9–10). Furthermore, they may reag-

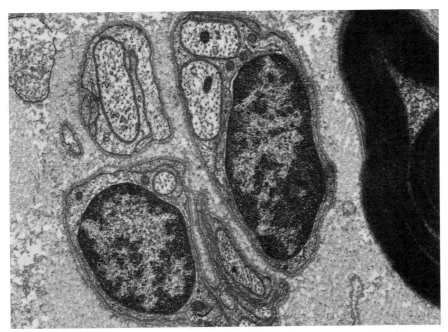

Figure 9-10. Electron micrograph showing unmyelinated nerve fibers. In contrast to myelinated fibers, several unmyelinated fibers may be invaginated into the cytoplasm of a single Schwann cell. For size comparison, note the large myelinated fiber to the right. ×20,000.

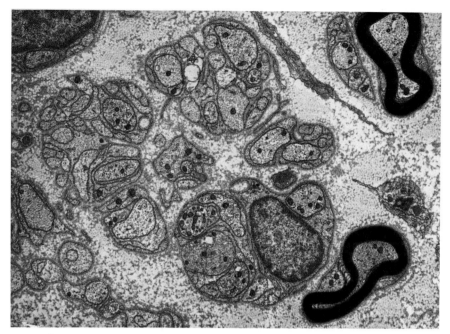

Figure 9-11. Electron micrograph showing regenerating nerve fibers in a sural nerve biopsy specimen from a patient with an axonal neuropathy. Note the basement membranes surrounding each cluster of regenerating axonal sprouts and Schwann cell processes. ×9000.

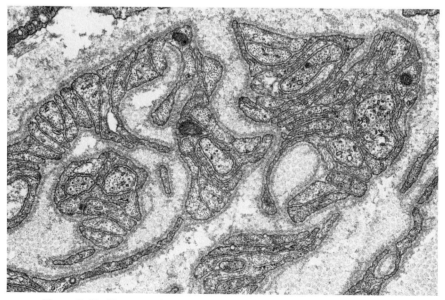

Figure 9-12. Electron micrograph showing a so-called band of Büngner. These bundles of Schwann cell processes and basement membranes result from axonal degeneration. ×30,000.

gregate as they move from the cytoplasm of one Schwann cell to another. Within the Schwann cell, the individual unmyelinated fibers are isolated from one another by tongues of Schwann cell cytoplasm. As in the case of myelinated fibers, the Schwann cells containing unmyelinated fibers are surrounded by a basement membrane. The Schwann cells may contain either myelinated fibers or unmyelinated fibers but not both. Normal unmyelinated fibers and their associated Schwann cell cytoplasm must be distinguished from regenerating nerve fibers and from bands of Büngner. The regenerating nerve fibers appear as clusters of small axonal sprouts and Schwann cell processes that are surrounded by a common basement membrane (Fig. 9–11). The basement membranes surrounding the clusters of regenerating axons apparently remain following the degeneration of preexisting myelinated nerve fibers. The so-called bands of Büngner (Fig. 9–12) are bundles of Schwann cell processes and basement membranes that remain following axonal degeneration. Ultimately these degenerate, unless invaded by regenerating axonal sprouts.

One must avoid attributing unwarranted significance to minor alterations in nerve specimens, especially sural nerve biopsy, from older individuals. Myelinated fibers show mild changes of segmental demyelination and axonal degeneration that become progressively more prominent with advancing age.[11] Similarly unmyelinated fibers may decrease in number and be replaced by stacks of Schwann cell profiles.[12]

References

1. Asbury AK, Johnson PC: Pathology of Peripheral Nerve. Philadelphia, Saunders, 1978.
2. Schaumburg HH, Spencer PS, Thomas PK: Disorders of Peripheral Nerves. Philadelphia, Davis, 1983.
3. Dyck PJ, Karnes J, Lais A, et al.: Pathologic alterations of the peripheral nervous system of humans. In Dyck PJ, Thomas PK, Lambert EH, Bunge R (eds): Peripheral Neuropathy, 2nd ed. Philadelphia, Saunders, 1984, Vol 1, pp 760–870.
4. Pollock M, Nukada H, Taylor P, et al.: Comparison between fascicular and whole sural nerve biopsy. Ann Neurol 13:65–68, 1983.
5. Kudo M, Griggs RC: Diagnostic usefulness of intramuscular nerve bundles. Arch Pathol Lab Med 106:355–359, 1982.
6. Low PA: Endoneurial fluid pressure and microenvironment of nerve. In Dyck PJ, Thomas PK, Lambert EH, Bunge R (eds): Peripheral Neuropathy, 2nd ed. Philadelphia, Saunders, 1984, Vol 1, pp 599–617.
7. Powell HC, Lampert PW: Peripheral neuropathy. In Rosenberg RN, Grossman RG, Schochet SS Jr, et al. (eds): The Clinical Neurosciences. New York, Churchill Livingstone, 1983, Vol 3, pp 325–362.
8. Bergouignan FX, Vital C: Occurence of Renaut's bodies in a peripheral nerve. Arch Pathol Lab Med 108:330–333, 1984.
9. Asbury AK: Renaut bodies. A forgotten endoneurial structure. J Neuropathol Exp Neurol 32:334–343, 1973.

10. Ortman JA, Sahenk Z, Mendell JR: The experimental production of Renaut bodies in response to mechanical stress. Neurology 32:A132, 1982.

11. Behse F, Carlsen F: Histology and ultrastructure of alterations in neuropathy. Muscle Nerve 1:368–374, 1978.

12. Ochoa J: Recognition of unmyelinated fiber disease: Morphological criteria. Muscle Nerve 1:375–387, 1978.

chapter 10

Inflammatory, Neoplastic, and Paraneoplastic Neuropathies

INFLAMMATORY NEUROPATHIES

For purposes of discussion in this chapter, the inflammatory neuropathies are divided into two broad, possibly overlapping groups. The first group comprises neuropathies that are considered by many workers to be mediated predominantly by immunologic mechanisms. This does not necessarily exclude the possibility that they are initiated by infectious agents. Among the disorders included in this category are the Guillain–Barré syndrome and the chronic inflammatory polyneuropathies. The second group of neuropathies include those caused by specific infectious agents such as leprosy and varicella–zoster. Even among the neuropathies caused by identified infectious agents, immunologic mechanisms may play a significant role in the pathogenesis of the clinical disorder.

GUILLAIN–BARRÉ SYNDROME (ACUTE INFLAMMATORY POLYNEUROPATHY)

The Guillain–Barré syndrome is a relatively common disorder typically manifested by the subacute evolution of an ascending paralysis. The disease is encountered throughout the world and affects individuals of all ages although it is somewhat more common in young adults. In approximately two thirds of the patients, there is a history of an antecedent acute illness 1 to 3 weeks previously. Most often, this is a "flulike" syndrome or gastrointestinal disorder. A wide variety of other antecedent illnesses or events have been described.

These have included cytomegalovirus and Epstein–Barr virus infections, mycoplasma infections, surgery, vaccinations, and other immunizations.[1] In recent years, the possibility of an association between the swine flu immunizations and the Guillain–Barré syndrome has received considerable attention.

The predominant clinical manifestation of the Guillain–Barré syndrome is progressive weakness. Most often the weakness begins in the legs. Later it may spread ("ascend") to involve the rest of the body. The weakness develops progressively over a period of time ranging from a few days to a few weeks. Although distal muscles are often more severely affected than the proximal muscles, involvement of the respiratory muscles is one of the most serious complications of the disease. Among the cranial nerves, the facial nerves are the most commonly affected. Characteristically, the deep tendon reflexes are markedly depressed even where there is minimal weakness. Objective sensory deficits are rarely demonstrable although sensory symptoms may be described. Many of the patients have prominent autonomic dysfunction manifested by unstable blood pressure and heart rate.

Examination of the cerebrospinal fluid characteristically reveals elevation of the protein content out of proportion to the cell count. Some authors have reported a less-favorable outcome among patients with normal protein levels during the initial phase of their illness.[2] In the majority of patients, electrodiagnostic studies show slowed nerve conduction velocities or even conduction block.

Nerve biopsies are rarely performed on these patients since their clinical manifestations are so characteristic. However, a small percentage of the patients die from this disease and these patients have provided much of our information regarding the underlying histopathology. The most characteristic morphologic feature is the presence of inflammatory cell infiltrates.[3] These range from scanty to abundant and are typically aggregated around small vessels within the peripheral nerves, spinal roots, and ganglia (Figs. 10–1 through 10–5). Many of the inflamed vessels appear to be small venules. Occasionally the endothelial cells are prominently swollen. The inflammatory cell infiltrates are composed predominantly of mononuclear cells including lymphocytes, transformed lymphocytes, macrophages, and occasional plasma cells. Rarely, small numbers of polymorphonuclear leukocytes also may be present. The involved nerves show mild to severe demyelination, some of which appears to be typical segmental demyelination. Other nerve fibers show axonal degeneration. The latter alteration is especially prominent in material obtained at autopsy. The affected nerves often appear diffusely hypercellular. This has been attributed to Schwann cell proliferation.

The changes in the distal peripheral nerves, spinal nerve roots, and ganglia are probably similar although involvement of the more proximal structures has been studied more extensively in autopsy material. There appear to be discrepancies between the morphologic findings and the typical clinical manifestations. Among the most striking are the equally severe involvement of motor and sensory roots and the prominent involvement of the dorsal root ganglia

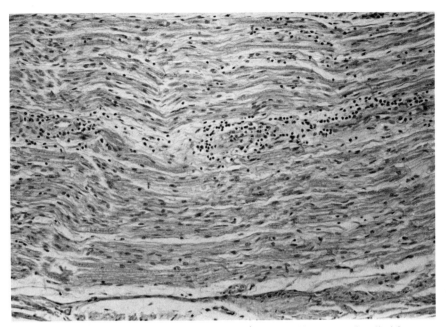

Figure 10-1. Sural nerve specimen from a 62-year-old woman who died 3 weeks after the onset of the Guillain–Barré syndrome. Scanty mononuclear cell infiltrates are present around blood vessels within the nerve. H&E, ×200.

despite the paucity of objective sensory findings on clinical examination. Another discrepancy is the frequency and severity of axonal degeneration in a disease that is regarded clinically as a predominantly demyelinative condition. The axonal degeneration has been attributed to foci of more severe inflammation in which there are polymorphonuclear leukocytes.[1] However, infiltrates of polymorphonuclear leukocytes are much less frequently encountered than axonal degeneration. The possibility of axonal injury from the lymphocytes deserves consideration. Regardless of the pathogenesis of the axonal injury, it is occasionally reflected in the spinal cord by chromatolysis of scattered anterior horn motor neurons and in the skeletal muscles by scattered foci of denervation. Rarely, small foci of inflammatory cells are seen in the skeletal muscles. Apparently these are extensions from affected intramuscular nerve twigs.

RELAPSING INFLAMMATORY NEUROPATHY

A small number of patients with acute inflammatory neuropathy experience relapses at intervals ranging from months to years after their initial illness.[4,5] The clinical features exhibited during the relapses are similar to those of the initial illness, however, the course of the disease may be somewhat more in-

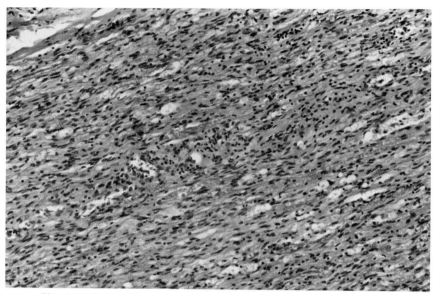

Figure 10-2. Dorsal root from a 61-year-old man who died from respiratory complications 3½ months after the onset of the Guillain–Barré syndrome. Note the perivascular mononuclear inflammatory cell infiltrates and widespread alterations in the myelin sheaths, reflecting demyelination. H&E, ×165.

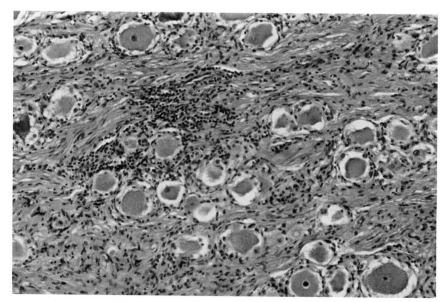

Figure 10-3. Dorsal root ganglion from same patient as in Figure 10-2. Note the mononuclear inflammatory cell infiltrates within the ganglion. H&E, ×165.

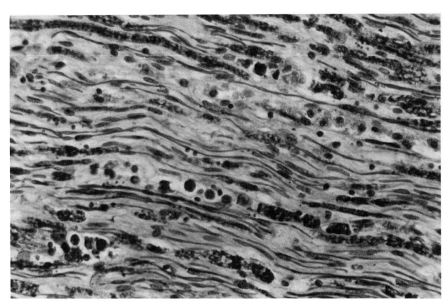

Figure 10-4. Spinal root from same patient as in Figure 10-2. These severe histologic alterations are the result of both demyelination and axonal degeneration. Trichrome, ×420.

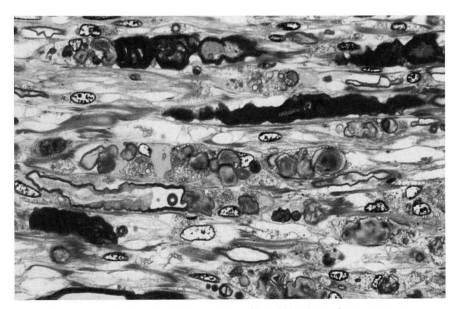

Figure 10-5. Epoxy-embedded section of brachial plexus from same patient as in Figure 10-1. Note the presence of lipid-laden macrophages and myelin ovoids. Toluidine blue, ×800.

dolent. The cerebrospinal fluid displays the expected elevated protein content and may also contain an increased number of mononuclear cells.

Histologic studies of peripheral nerves from these patients have shown morphologic features that are similar to the acute disease, e.g., mononuclear inflammatory cell infiltrates and demyelination. In addition, there may be evidence of remyelination in the form of shortened internodes that are invested in thin myelin sheaths and, rarely, even small onion bulb formations.

CHRONIC INFLAMMATORY NEUROPATHY

This is a relatively uncommon form of inflammatory neuropathy that is not clearly distinguished from relapsing inflammatory neuropathy. Although this disease is thought to be mediated by immunologic mechanisms, an antecedent illness has been documented in only a small proportion of the affected individuals.[6] The disease pursues a progressive course that is variable in nature and may extend over many years. The cerebrospinal fluid shows elevation of the protein content out of proportion to the cell count. Electrodiagnostic studies show evidence of demyelination.

Histologic studies on these patients have shown endoneurial edema, inflammation, demyelination, and remyelination of varying degrees. The inflammatory cell infiltrates are composed of mononuclear cells but may be much less prominent than in cases of acute or relapsing inflammatory neuropathy. The repeated episodes of demyelination and remyelination are often reflected by the presence of numerous onion bulbs. In some patients, these are quite large and readily seen in paraffin-embedded sections (Figs. 10-6 and 10-7). In other patients, even when they are less conspicuous, they are readily demonstrated in epoxy-embedded sections (Fig. 10-8). The intervening endoneurial tissue often contains an increased number of fibroblasts and amorphous granular material.

By electron microscopy, the onion bulbs appear as myelinated or remyelinated axons surrounded by variable numbers of concentric lamellae composed of Schwann cell processes. These are separated by layers of collagen in which most of the fibrils are oriented longitudinally. The onion bulbs are indicative of the repeated episodes of demyelination and remyelination but are not diagnostic of any specific disorder.

LEPROSY

Although rare in the United States, leprosy is a common disease and a very important cause of peripheral neuropathy in many parts of the world.[7,8] Epidemiologic studies have estimated that there are currently 12 to 15 million cases of leprosy worldwide. The disease is more common in tropical and subtropical areas, especially parts of Asia, Africa, and South America.

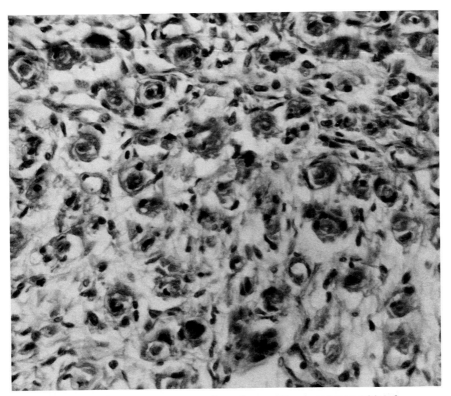

Figure 10-6. Peripheral nerve specimen from a 74-year-old man with a 3-year history of chronic inflammatory polyneuropathy. His cerebrospinal fluid protein content was 218 mg/dl shortly before his death. Although no inflammatory cell infiltrates are present, there is prominent endoneurial edema and numerous onion bulb formations. Trichrome, ×410.

The disease is caused by infection with *Mycobacterium leprae,* an organism this is morphologically similar to *Mycobacterium tuberculosis* but less acid-fast. This is an important consideration in the histologic diagnosis of leprosy since the organisms are not reliably demonstrated by many of the usual staining techniques, e.g., the Ziehl–Neelsen stain, employed for the detection of tubercle baccili. Many authors find the Fite–Faraco method more dependable.[9]

The organisms usually enter through the skin, although in some cases infection may occur through the mucous membranes of the mouth and upper respiratory tract. Only a small proportion of the population is thought to be susceptible to the infection. The disease has a prolonged incubation period estimated to be 3 to 5 years. The bacteria proliferate slowly and have a predilection to invade peripheral nerves. The subsequent course and clinical manifestations of the disease are determined largely by the degree of cell-mediated immunoresponsiveness of the host. At least four different patterns of disease are widely recognized.

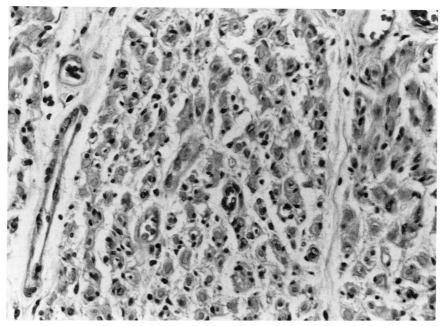

Figure 10-7. Spinal root from a 51-year-old man with a 6-year history of chronic inflammatory polyneuropathy. The cerebrospinal fluid protein content was 132 mg/dl shortly before his death. Note the numerous onion bulb formations. H&E, ×430.

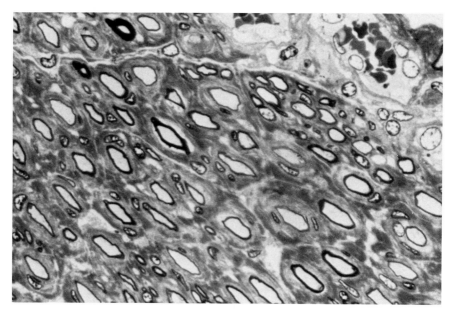

Figure 10-8. Chronic inflammatory polyneuropathy, same patient as in Figure 10-7. The onion bulb formations are even more conspicuous in this epoxy-embedded section of a spinal nerve root. Toluidine blue, ×700.

Indeterminate leprosy is thought to be a very early form of the disease and is manifested by a single erythematous or hypopigmented papule or macule in which there is altered sensation. Biopsy specimens disclose mononuclear cell infiltrates about skin appendages, cutaneous nerves, and vessels. The organisms are sparse, and when demonstrable are most apt to be found in the cutaneous nerve twigs. Indeterminate leprosy can heal, with or without treatment, or can progress to one of the other forms of the disease.

Tuberculoid leprosy is associated with a high degree of immunoresponsiveness that limits the proliferation and dissemination of the organisms. This form of the disease is manifested by one or a few sharply demarcated hypopigmented areas in which there is reduced sensation. The lesions are asymmetrically distributed and are found most often on the extensor surfaces of the extremities, buttocks, and face. Biopsy specimens disclose granulomas that contain epithelioid cells, giant cells, and mononuclear inflammatory cells. The granulomas characteristically extend up to the basal layer of the skin. Dermal and subcutaneous nerves may be severely involved or destroyed by caseation necrosis. Organisms are sparse, and when demonstrable, are most apt to be found in the remnants of the peripheral nerves.

Lepromatous leprosy is associated with a low degree of host immunoresponsiveness and hematogenous dissemination of the organisms.[9,10] This form of the disease is manifested by erythematous or hypopigmented macules, papules, and nodules. The lesions may be widely scattered and have a predilection for the cooler portions of the body. Initially, sensation may be preserved within the skin lesions. Later, however, widespread sensory loss ensues in the distal and cooler portions of the body. Biopsy specimens disclose heavy histiocytic infiltrates accompanied by lesser numbers of other mononuclear inflammatory cells within the dermis. The infiltrates are especially prominent about skin appendages, nerve twigs (Fig. 10-9), and blood vessels. However, the inflammatory cell infiltrates typically spare a thin zone immediately beneath the epidermis. Large numbers of organisms can be demonstrated readily within the cytoplasm of the dermal histiocytes. Bacilli can also be demonstrated in Schwann cells of nerves underlying the skin lesions. Involvement of various visceral organs has been demonstrated in patients with lepromatous leprosy.

Dimorphous or borderline leprosy is associated with an intermediate degree of host immunoresponsiveness. This form of the disease is characterized clinically and pathologically by a variable admixture of the features encountered in both tuberculoid and lepromatous leprosy.

SARCOIDOSIS

Sarcoidosis is a systemic granulomatous disorder of unknown etiology and pathogenesis. On a worldwide basis, it is much less common than leprosy but is more frequently encountered in this country. Neurologic involvement has been estimated to occur in only about 5 percent of patients and is due pre-

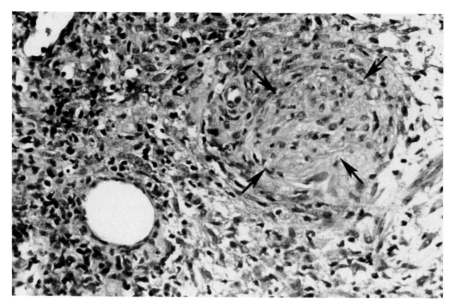

Figure 10-9. Lepromatous leprosy. Note the small dermal nerve *(arrows)* that is partially surrounded by an inflammatory cell infiltrate which includes numerous foamy histiocytes. H&E, ×400.

dominantly to granulomatous basal meningitis with involvement of adjacent structures.[11] Hypothalamic dysfunction, facial paralysis, and visual impairment are relatively common. However, if cranial nerve and spinal root lesions are excluded, symptomatic involvement of the peripheral nervous system is rare. Nevertheless, both mononeuropathy multiplex and symmetrical polyneuropathies have been reported.[12,13] Histologic studies are limited but sural nerve biopsy specimens have shown axonal degeneration and segmental demyelination in association with typical noncaseating granulomas. The granulomas were within the endoneurium as well as in the nerve ensheathments. Panangiitis, similar to the vascular involvement in the central nervous system, was prominent in the patient reported by Oh.[12] The peripheral nerve dysfunction has been attributed to both mechanical compression and vascular insufficiency.

HERPES ZOSTER

Herpes zoster is a relatively common disorder that has been recognized for centuries. The disease is thought to result from the reactivation of a latent varicella–zoster infection of various sensory ganglia with development of a vesicular eruption in the corresponding area of cutaneous innervation. Most commonly these are thoracic dermatomes or areas of trigeminal innervation. The appearance of the cutaneous vesicles is often preceded by pain or other abnormal sensations.

Histologically, the skin lesions are typical viral vesicles with acantholysis and intranuclear inclusions in enlarged epithelial cells. Abnormalities in the corresponding sensory ganglia have long been recognized. In a classic study, Head and Campbell[14] reported ganglia to be hemorrhagic and necrotic when examined during the acute stages of the disease. Months to years later, ganglia from severely affected individuals are shrunken and discolored. Rarely, intranuclear inclusions can be seen by light microscopy in the ganglion cells and accompanying satellite cells.[15] More often one merely sees infiltrates of mononuclear inflammatory cells. The virus can be demonstrated by electron microscopy and immunocytologic techniques, and has been isolated from dorsal root ganglia.[16]

VASCULITIC NEUROPATHIES

Vasculitis is an integral part of the pathologic alterations encountered in many of the so-called collagen vascular diseases. Medium and small vessels including the vasa nervorum are affected selectively. Thus peripheral neuropathy is not an unexpected finding in many of these conditions. Most commonly, the nerve involvement is manifested as a mononeuropathy multiplex, however, a distal symmetrical polyneuropathy can be encountered in some patients.

Peripheral neuropathy is most apt to be encountered among patients with the polyarteritis nodosa group of necrotizing vasculitides. This category includes classical polyarteritis nodosa, allergic granulomatosis, hypersensitivity vasculitis, and various overlapping syndromes.[17] These diseases appear to be initiated by immune complexes deposited in blood vessel walls. Complement components are activated and attract polymorphonuclear leukocytes. The subsequent vascular damage is produced, at least in part, by the release of lysosomal enzymes from the polymorphonuclear leukocytes. In recent years, hepatitis B antigenemia has become recognized as an important predisposing condition.[18] Similar lesions have also been associated with cryoglobulinemia and amphetamine abuse.[19]

About two thirds of patients with polyarteritis nodosa have peripheral neuropathies at some time during the course of their illness. The neuropathy may even be the initial manifestation of the disease. An even higher proportion have peripheral nerve lesions that can be demonstrated histologically.[20] The lesions are found predominantly in the epineurial vessels; the endoneurial vessels tend to be spared. When the lesions are acute, the vessel walls may show foci of fibrinoid necrosis. The mural necrosis is accompanied by varying proportions of polymorphonuclear leukocytes, including occasional eosinophils and mononuclear inflammatory cells (Figs. 10–10 and 10–11). Occasionally there may be small hemorrhages. During the healing stages, the vessels may show mural

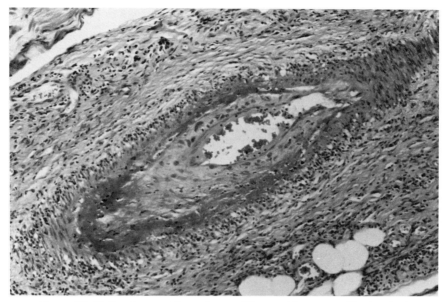

Figure 10-10. Sural nerve biopsy from a 55-year-old woman with classical polyarteritis. The necrotizing arteritis is seen in an epineurial arteriole. H&E, ×220.

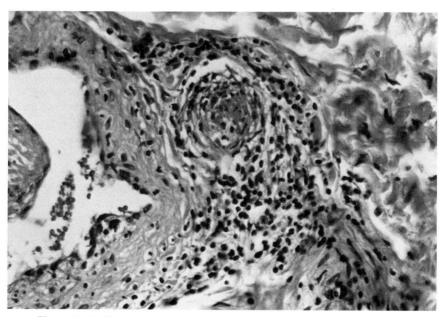

Figure 10-11. Sural nerve biopsy specimen from a 40-year-old man with polyarteritis manifested by recent onset of myalgias, hypertension, and renal failure. The affected arteriole is within the epineurial connective tissue. H&E, ×400.

fibrosis with minimal inflammation. Only the foci of mural necrosis are considered diagnostic. The nerve itself generally shows patchy areas of injury consisting of both axonal degeneration and segmental demyelination. The central portions of the nerve fascicles may be more severely affected. True infarcts are rarely if ever encountered. Observations in patients with rheumatoid vasculitis have prompted Dyck et al.[21] to suggest that the vasculitic damage is maximal in watershed areas of less abundant perfusion.

At least some of the neuropathies associated with rheumatoid disease[21,22] and Sjögren's syndrome[22] are due to necrotizing vasculitides that are histologically indistinguishable from polyarteritis. Necrotizing vasculitis also may be the basis for the neuropathy in at least some patients with systemic lupus erythematosus. In others, the neuropathy is demyelinative.[23]

NEOPLASTIC AND PARANEOPLASTIC NEUROPATHIES

Direct Neoplastic Involvement of the Peripheral Nerves

Peripheral nerves give rise to a variety of primary neoplasms, most of which are derived from Schwann cells. Although they may pose difficult diagnostic problems, they are more appropriately discussed in books and atlases on tumor pathology.[24] Peripheral nerves are also involved, both directly and indirectly by various metastatic and hematogenous neoplasms. Direct compression of spinal nerves and nerve roots is commonly encountered in patients with metastatic carcinoma, lymphoma, and myeloma. These are predominantly mechanical injuries that result from a combination of epidural metastases, vertebral metastases, and fractures complicating the spinal metastases. The peripheral nerve lesions are often accompanied by and overshadowed by compression of the spinal cord. Cranial nerves and spinal nerve roots are commonly involved in association with meningeal carcinomatosis (Fig. 10–12) and central nervous system leukemia (Fig. 10–13). More localized neuropathies may result from neoplastic involvement of the brachial and lumbosacral plexi. The brachial plexi are often involved in carcinoma of the lung and breast, while the lumbosacral plexi are commonly affected in retroperitoneal and pelvic neoplasms including carcinoma of the prostate and cervix, and lymphomas. Although many carcinomas give rise to local epineurial metastases, distant hematogenous metastases are very rare. By contrast, lymphomas and leukemias may produce regionally, more diffuse involvement of peripheral nerves. These may mimic other types of peripheral neuropathies.

Indirect Neoplastic Involvement of the Peripheral Nerves

Although relatively rare, several clinical syndromes have been attributed to the remote effects of malignancies on the peripheral nervous system.[25-27] A mixed motor and sensory neuropathy may be encountered in association with various

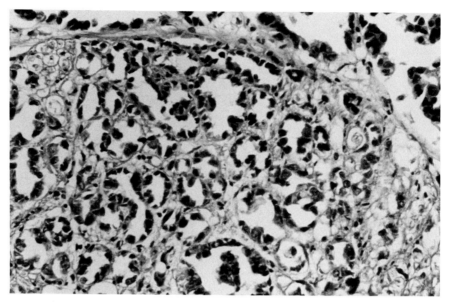

Figure 10-12. Dorsal spinal root involvement in association with meningeal carcinomatosis from adenocarcinoma of the lung. H&E, ×350.

types of carcinoma, especially carcinomas of the lung, breast, and gastrointestinal tract. These patients have weakness and impairment to varying degrees of all sensory modalities. The lower extremities tend to be more severely affected than the upper extremities. Histologic studies of peripheral nerve specimens have shown predominantly axonal degeneration with secondary demyelination. Although even less common than in association with carcinomas, similar if not identical neuropathies have been described in patients with lymphomas and myeloma.

A rare but clinically distinctive sensory neuropathy has also been delineated.[25-27] This disorder occurs predominantly in patients with oat cell carcinoma of the lung although it has been seen in association with other types of carcinoma and lymphomas. The neuropathy may develop months before the neoplasm is otherwise detected. The neuropathy is subacute in course but is often quite severe. It is manifested by pain, paresthesias, and loss of position sense. Patients with this disorder often have an elevated cerebrospinal fluid protein content.

Histopathologic studies on patients with this disorder have revealed a ganglioradiculopathy.[27] The dorsal root ganglia show prominent degenerative changes with loss of ganglion cells, clusters of residual satellite cells, and variably severe lymphoplasmocytic inflammatory cell infiltrates. The dorsal roots also show degenerative changes and may be infiltrated by mononuclear inflam-

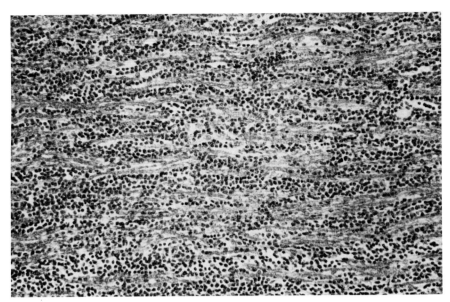

Figure 10-13. Oculomotor nerve involvement in a 38-year-old woman with acute lymphocytic leukemia. H&E, ×220.

matory cells. The posterior columns of the spinal cord are demyelinated. Peripheral nerve specimens generally show severe loss of sensory nerve fibers. This may be especially severe in a predominantly sensory nerve such as the sural nerve but the changes by themselves are not morphologically distinctive.

Mononeuritis multiplex secondary to vasculitis has been reported in three patients prior to diagnosis of underlying malignancies.[28] Two of these patients were subsequently found to have carcinomatous sensory neuropathy secondary to oat cell carcinomas of the lung and the third was found to have lymphoma and later, liposarcoma. These authors suggested that this vasculitis, largely limited to the peripheral nervous system, represented still another type of neuropathy arising as a remote effect of the malignancies.

Despite extensive investigations, the pathogenesis of these neuropathies developing in association with various neoplasms remains unclear. Activation of latent viral infections, toxins secreted by the neoplasms, deficiency states, and immunologic abnormalities have been proposed as possible mechanisms. An immunologic mechanism has received support from a recent study of sural nerve specimens from patients with polyneuropathies associated with various types of carcinomas and Hodgkin's disease.[29] These authors found deposits of immunoglobulin M and complement components on the perineurium and around endoneurial capillaries in the patients with neuropathy, but not in their control patients with malignancies without a neuropathy.

NEUROPATHIES ASSOCIATED WITH
ABNORMAL GLOBULIN PRODUCTION

In recent years, there has been increased recognition of polyneuropathies in association with abnormal globulin production.[30] In addition to compressive lesions resulting from local involvement of the vertebral column and skull, myeloma is responsible for causing occasional cases of polyneuropathy. Among patients with typical myeloma, this is a relatively rare complication and is most often a mixed sensory and motor neuropathy. Histologically, nerve specimens from these individuals are characterized predominantly by axonal degeneration with only mild, probably secondary, demyelination. Despite prior reports to the contrary, amyloid is encountered relatively infrequently in nerve biopsy specimens from these patients. By contrast, patients with the rarer osteosclerotic form of myeloma have a much higher prevalence of peripheral nerve involvement.[31,32] This is often manifested predominantly as a motor neuropathy and may be evident months before their myeloma is diagnosed. Morphologic studies on nerve specimens from these patients have demonstrated more extensive demyelination accompanied by mild mononuclear cell infiltrates.

Macroglobulinemia is characterized by the excessive production of immunoglobulin M (IgM), a large 19S carbohydrate-containing molecule. This may occur in association with various lymphoplasmocytic neoplasms, occasional nonhematopoietic neoplasms, and certain nonneoplastic conditions. Patients with macroglobulinemia often develop peripheral neuropathies, and even when due to neoplastic causes, these may be the initial manifestation of their disease. The neuropathies are most often mixed sensory and motor neuropathies[33] although some cases of nearly pure motor neuropathy have been described.[34] Histologic studies on nerve biopsy specimens have revealed predominantly demyelination with mild axonal degeneration. Rare "onion bulb" formations reflecting remyelination also may be seen. These nerve fiber abnormalities may be accompanied by scanty infiltrates of mononuclear cells including lymphocytes and plasma cells.[33,35,36] Small deposits of IgM that appear as amorphous material that stains positively with the PAS reaction may be encountered within the endoneurium and perineurium and about small blood vessels. The vessel walls may be thickened as the result of endothelial proliferation.[37] Ultrastructurally, several of these patients have shown striking separation of myelin lamellae.[36–39] Occasionally, amyloid has been seen in peripheral nerves from individuals with macroglobulinemia.[39] Similar histologic changes have also been seen in patients with polyneuropathies associated with benign immunoglobulin G (IgG) gammopathies.[30]

Cryoglobulinemia is characterized by the presence of serum globulins that precipitate upon cooling and redissolve upon warming to body temperature. These may be found in patients with various lymphoplasmocytic neoplasms and nonhematopoietic neoplasms, and in association with various infections and collagen-vascular diseases. Some of these patients also have peripheral neuropathy, either a mixed sensory and motor polyneuropathy or mononeuropathy multiplex. Histologic studies have shown both demyelination and axonal degeneration. One patient was further characterized ultrastructurally by the presence of osmiophilic material in the endoneurium and blood vessels. This material was composed of closely packed tubular aggregates similar to cryoglobulin.[40] Other patients have shown necrotizing vasculitis and perineurial inflammatory cell infiltrates.[41,42]

AMYLOID NEUROPATHY

Amyloid is a proteinaceous material that can be derived from a number of different precursor compounds.[43] Immunoglobulin light-chain components are the precursors for the amyloid encountered in primary amyloidosis and in association with the various dysproteinemic states, while the so-called "SAA protein" is the precursor for the amyloid seen in secondary or reactive systemic amyloidosis. The precursor for the amyloid found in the hereditary amyloid neuropathies is thought to be prealbumin.[44,45] Despite the varied pathogenesis, all forms of amyloid have a fibrillar ultrastructure and show an apple-green birefringence color when viewed with polarized light after staining with Congo Red. The latter features are attributed to the unusual beta-pleated sheet molecular structure that is shared by all forms of amyloid.

Amyloid neuropathy may be encountered in patients with primary amyloidosis, in association with plasma cell dyscrasias and in the various forms of hereditary amyloid neuropathy. Amyloid neuropathy is rarely if ever the result of so-called secondary or reactive systemic amyloidosis. As previously indicated, only some of the neuropathies associated with plasma cell dyscrasias can be attributed to amyloid deposition in and about peripheral nerves.

The clinical manifestations of amyloid neuropathy are varied. Patients with nonhereditary amyloid neuropathy often have a painful distal polyneuropathy with prominent sensory involvement.[46] Loss of pain and temperature perception is frequently more severe than loss of vibration and position sense. Autonomic dysfunction, manifested by orthostatic hypotension, gastrointestinal disturbances, impaired bladder function, and decreased sweating, is common. A carpal tunnel syndrome, due to amyloid deposition in the flexor retinaculum, is commonly found in patients with all forms of amyloid neuropathy.[47] The hereditary amyloid neuropathies are relatively rare autosomal-dominant disorders that are characterized by their patterns of clinical involvement.[48] At least four types can be distinguished. The so-called "Portuguese" form, which is also found in other countries, appears to be the most prevalent and has been studied the most extensively.[49]

Histopathologic studies on specimens from patients with amyloid neuropathy disclose focal or diffuse deposits of amyloid within the endoneurium (Fig. 10–14) and within the walls of the vasa nervorum. The nerve fibers show axonal degeneration with especially severe loss of small myelinated and unmyelinated nerve fibers. Dorsal root and sympathetic ganglia are often heavily

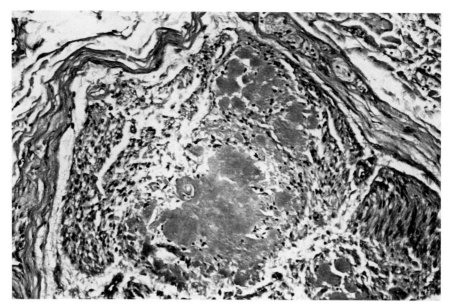

Figure 10-14. Endoneurial amyloid deposits in a 72-year-old man with primary amyloidosis. Trichrome, ×200.

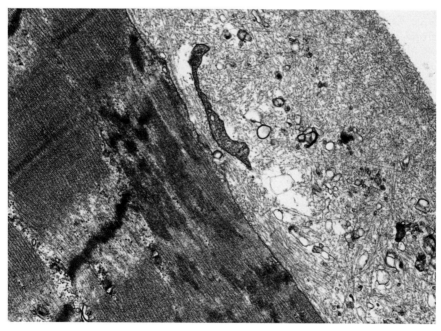

Figure 10-15. Electron micrograph of a skeletal muscle biopsy specimen from a 60-year-old woman with primary amyloidosis and proximal upper-extremity weakness. Note the endomysial deposits of amyloid fibrils. ×30,000.

infiltrated with amyloid. Connective tissue removed during surgical decompression of entrapment neuropathies may reveal amyloid, even in the absence of other evidence of amyloid neuropathy.[50] As in other tissues, amyloid stains red with H&E, green with trichrome, and red with PAS techniques. Identification of the amyloid is best accomplished by the use of the Congo Red stain followed by demonstration of the characteristic apple-green birefringence color with polarized light. The sections should be carefully decolorized since spurious staining can result from retention of excess stain.[51] If desired, further confirmation can be achieved by electron microscopy. This will reveal a feltwork of straight fibrils each measuring approximately 10 nm in diameter (Fig. 10–15).

The basis for the nerve dysfunction in amyloid neuropathy remains uncertain. Direct mechanical compression by the deposits of amyloid and ischemia secondary to deposits of amyloid within vasa nervorum, are among the major considerations. Alternatively, it has been suggested that the nerves undergo degeneration because of an underlying metabolic derangement and the amyloid deposits are merely an epiphenomenon. In some patients, the neuromuscular complications of amyloidosis include weakness and pseudohypertrophy of muscles.[52,53] Histopathologic studies on these patients have revealed deposits of amyloid within the endomysial connective tissue (Fig. 10–15) as well as in nerves and blood vessels. Although the deposits are outside of the sarcolemma, it has been suggested that the amyloid interferes with the normal propagation of action potentials along the surface of the muscle fibers.[53]

References

1. Arnason BGW: Acute inflammatory demyelinating polyradiculoneuropathies. In Dyck PJ, Thomas PK, Lambert EH, Bunge R (eds): Peripheral Neuropathy. Philadelphia, Saunders, 1984, Vol 2, pp 2050–2100.
2. Asbury AK: Diagnostic considerations in Guillain–Barré syndrome. Ann Neurol 9 (Suppl):1–5, 1981.
3. Asbury AK, Arnason BG, Adams RD: The inflammatory lesion in idiopathic polyneuritis: Its role in pathogenesis. Medicine 48:173–215, 1969.
4. Borit A, Altrocchi PH: Recurrent polyneuropathy and neurolymphomatosis. Arch Neurol 24:40–49, 1971.
5. Prineas JW, McLeod JG: Chronic relapsing polyneuritis. J Neurol Sci 27:427–458, 1976.
6. Dyck PJ, Lais AC, Bastron JA, et al.: Chronic inflammatory polyradiculoneuropathy. Mayo Clinic Proc 50:621–637, 1975.
7. Dastur DK: The nervous system in leprosy. In Goldensohn ES, Appel SH (eds): Scientific Approaches to Clinical Neurology. New York, Lea & Febiger, 1977, Vol 2, pp 1456–1493.
8. Binford CH, Meyers WM, Walsh GP: Leprosy. JAMA 247:2283–2292, 1982.
9. Lawrence C, Schreiber AJ: Leprosy's footprints in bone-marrow histiocytes. N Engl J Med 300:834–835, 1979.

10. Drutz DJ, Chen TSN, Lu WH: The continuous bacteremia of lepromatous leprosy. N Engl J Med 287:159–164, 1972.
11. Delaney P: Neurological manifestations in sarcoidosis. Review of the literature, with a report of 23 cases. Ann Intern Med 87:336–345, 1977.
12. Oh SJ: Sarcoid polyneuropathy: A histologically proved case. Ann Neurol 7:178–181, 1980.
13. Nemni R, Galassi G, Cohen M, et al.: Symmetric sarcoid polyneuropathy: Analysis of a sural nerve biopsy. Neurology 31:1217–1223, 1981.
14. Head H, Campbell AW: The pathology of herpes zoster and its bearing on sensory localization. Brain 23:353–523, 1900.
15. Ghatak NR, Zimmerman HM: Spinal ganglion in herpes zoster. A light and electron microscopic study. Arch Pathol 95:411–415, 1973.
16. Bastian FO, Rabson AS, Yee CL, Tralka TS: Herpesvirus varicellae. Isolated from human dorsal root ganglia. Arch Pathol 97:331–333, 1974.
17. Fauci AS, Haynes BF, Katz P: The spectrum of vasculitis. Clinical, pathological, immunologic, and therapeutic considerations. Ann Intern Med 89:660–676, 1978.
18. Sergent JS, Lockshin MD, Christain CL, Gocke DJ: Vasculitis with hepatitis B antigenemia: Long-term observations in nine patients. Medicine 55:1–18, 1976.
19. Citron BP, Halpern M, McCarron M, et al.: Necrotizing angiitis in drug addicts. N Engl J Med 283:1003–1011, 1970.
20. Lovshin LL, Kernohan JW: Peripheral neuritis in periarteritis nodosa: A clinicopathologic study. Arch Intern Med 82:321–338, 1948.
21. Dyck PJ, Conn DL, Okazaki H: Necrotizing angiopathic neuropathy: Three dimensional morphology of fiber degeneration related to sites of occluded vessels. Mayo Clin Proc 47:461–475, 1972.
22. Peyronnard JM, Charron L, Beaudet F, Couture F: Vasculitis neuropathy in rheumatoid disease and Sjögren syndrome. Neurology 32:839–845, 1982.
23. Rechthand E, Cornblath DR, Stern BJ, Meyerhoff JD: Chronic demyelinating polyneuropathy in systemic lupus erythematosus. Neurology 34:1375–1377, 1984.
24. Harkin JC, Reed RJ: Tumors of the peripheral nervous system. In Atlas of Tumor Pathology. Second Series, Fascicle 3. Washington, D.C., Armed Forces Institute of Pathology, 1969.
25. Henson RA, Urich H: Cancer and the Nervous System. Oxford, Blackwell, 1982, pp 368–405.
26. McLeod JG: Carcinomatous neuropathy. In Dyck PJ, Thomas PK, Lambert EH, Bunge R (eds): Peripheral Neuropathy. Philadelphia, Saunders, 1984, Vol 2, pp 2180–2191.
27. Horwich MS, Cho L, Porro RS, Posner JB: Subacute sensory neuropathy: A remote effect of carcinoma. Ann Neurol 2:7–19, 1977.
28. Johnson PC, Rolak LA, Hamilton RH, Laguna JF: Paraneoplastic vasculitis of nerve: A remote effect of cancer. Ann Neurol 5:437–444, 1979.
29. Ongerboer de Visser BW, Feltkamp-Vroom TM, Feltkamp CA: Sural nerve immune deposits in polyneuropathy as a remote effect of malignancy. Ann Neurol 14:261–266, 1983.
30. Kelly JJ Jr: Peripheral neuropathies associated with monoclonal proteins: A clinical review. Muscle Nerve 8:138–150, 1985.
31. Ohi T, Kyle RA, Dyck PJ: Axonal attenuation and secondary segmental demyelination in myeloma neuropathies. Ann Neurol 17:255–261, 1985.
32. Kelly JJ Jr, Kyle RA, Miles JM, Dyck PJ: Osteosclerotic myeloma and peripheral neuropathy. Neurology 33:202–210, 1983.

33. Sparr FW: Paraproteinaemias and multiple myeloma. In Vinken PJ, Bruyn GE (eds): Handbook of Clinical Neurology, Amsterdam, North-Holland, 1980, Vol 39, pp 131–179.

34. Rowland LP, Defendini R, Sherman WH, et al.: Macroglobulinemia with peripheral neuropathy simulating motor neuron disease. Ann Neurol 11:532–536, 1982.

35. Nemni R, Galassi G, Latov N, et al.: Polyneuropathy in non-malignant IgM plasma cell dyscrasia: A morphological study. Ann Neurol 14:43–54, 1983.

36. Julien J, Vital C, Vallat JM, et al.: Chronic demyelinating neuropathy with IgM-producing lymphocytes in peripheral nerve and delayed appearance of "benign" monoclonal gammopathy. Neurology 34:1387–1389, 1984.

37. Powell HC, Rodriguez M, Hughes AC: Microangiopathy of vasa nervorum in dysglobulinemic neuropathy. Ann Neurol 15:386–394, 1984.

38. Melmed C, Frial D, Duncan I, et al.: Peripheral neuropathy with IgM kappa monoclonal immunoglobulin directed against myelin-associated glycoprotein. Neurology 33:1397–1405, 1983.

39. Julien J, Vital C, Vallat JM, et al.: IgM demyelinative neuropathy with amyloidosis and biclonal gammopathy. Ann Neurol 15:395–399, 1984.

40. Vallat JM, Desproges-Gotteron R, Leboutet MJ, et al.: Cryoglobulinemic neuropathy: A pathological study. Ann Neurol 8:179–185, 1980.

41. Chad D, Pariser K, Bradley WG, et al.: The pathogenesis of cryoglobulinemia neuropathy. Neurology 32:725–729, 1982.

42. Konishi T, Saida K, Ohnishi A, Nishitani H: Perineuritis in mononeuropathy multiplex with cryoglobulinemia. Muscle Nerve 5:173–177, 1982.

43. Glenner GG: Amyloid deposits and amyloidosis. The β-fibrilloses. N Engl J Med 302:1283–1292, 1980; 302:1333–1343, 1980.

44. Costa PP, Figueira AS, Bravo FR: Amyloid fibril protein related to prealbumin in familial amyloid polyneuropathy. Proc Natl Acad Sci 75:4499–4503, 1978.

45. Dalakas MC, Engel WK: Amyloid in hereditary amyloid polyneuropathy is related to prealbumin. Arch Neurol 38:420–422, 1981.

46. Kelly JJ Jr, Kyle RA, O'Brien PC, Dyck PJ: The natural history of peripheral neuropathy in primary systemic amyloidosis. Ann Neurol 6:1–7, 1979.

47. Asbury AK, Johnson PC: Pathology of Peripheral Nerve. Philadelphia, Saunders, 1978, pp 148–155.

48. Cohen AS, Rubinow A: Amyloid neuropathy. In Dyck PJ, Thomas PK, Lambert E, Bunge R (eds): Peripheral Neuropathy. Philadelphia, Saunders, 1984, Vol 2, pp 1866–1898.

49. Said G, Ropert A, Faux N: Length-dependent degeneration of fibers in Portuguese amyloid polyneuropathy: A clinicopathologic study. Neurology 34:1025–1032, 1984.

50. Bastian FD: Amyloidosis and the carpal tunnel syndrome. Am J Clin Pathol 61:711–717, 1974.

51. Carson FL, Kingsley WB: Nonamyloid green birefringence following Congo Red staining. Arch Pathol Lab Med 104:333–335, 1980.

52. Whitaker JN, Hashimoto K, Quinones M: Skeletal muscle pseudohypertrophy in amyloidosis. Neurology 27:47–54, 1977.

53. Ringel SP, Claman HN: Amyloid-associated muscle pseudohypertrophy. Arch Neurol 39:413–417, 1982.

chapter 11

Systemic, Metabolic, and Toxic Neuropathies

DIABETIC NEUROPATHIES

In clinical practice, diabetes mellitus is one of the most common causes of peripheral neuropathies.[1] Nevertheless, the exact incidence of this complication is difficult to ascertain. The reported prevalence figures have varied widely, depending upon the criteria employed for diagnosing the presence of neuropathy. Nevertheless, most authors agree that the prevalence of the neuropathy increases with the duration of the disease. Neuropathy is generally regarded as uncommon in children with diabetes but may be present in over half of the adults who are over age 40. Despite extensive investigations in patients and experimental animals, the pathogenesis of the various diabetic neuropathies remains controversial.[2,3]

The diabetic neuropathies are commonly classified in two broad categories, the symmetrical polyneuropathies and the focal and multifocal neuropathies.[1] Autonomic neuropathy is included in the first category, while the isolated cranial nerve palsies and the mononeuropathies involving various large peripheral nerves are included in the second category. The symmetrical polyneuropathies are the more commonly encountered disorders and are often attributed to a diffuse metabolic disturbance secondary to chronic hyperglycemia.[3] These neuropathies range from clinically asymptomatic to severe. The manifestations are often predominantly sensory, in which a spectrum of "small-fiber," "large-fiber," and mixed patterns[4] have been delineated. The symmetrical polyneuropathies tend to affect the legs and feet more than the arms and are commonly accompanied by autonomic dysfunction. They may be accompanied by muscle wasting.

The focal and multifocal neuropathies are much less common and are more often attributed to vascular involvement. Among the cranial nerve palsies, oculomotor nerve involvement with pupillary sparing is an especially common complication of diabetes. Diabetes has also been implicated in a relatively high percentage of mononeuropathies involving the femoral nerve.[5] Proximal motor neuropathy, formerly designated as diabetic amyotrophy, is regarded by some authors[1] as another category of the focal and multifocal neuropathies, while others[3] feel that it is more closely related to the metabolic polyneuropathies.

Pathologic studies on peripheral nerves from patients with the diabetic polyneuropathies have shown both segmental demyelination and axonal degeneration. Although axonal degeneration is the predominant alteration, some specimens have shown prominent segmental demyelination and even onion bulb formations reflecting remyelination.[6,7] The significance of these dual patterns of injury remains unclear. Dyck et al.,[8] encountered segmental demyelination and remyelination in untreated asymptomatic patients, both segmental demyelination and axonal degeneration in untreated symptomatic patients, and predominantly axonal degeneration in treated patients with long-standing neuropathy. However, the segmental demyelination was not accompanied by or was secondary to axonal atrophy, as seen in experimental diabetic neuropathy induced with streptozotocin.[9] Another feature that has been observed in diabetic polyneuropathy is thickening of basement membranes in the peripheral nerves and dorsal root ganglia.[10,11] However, none of these changes are sufficiently distinctive to be of diagnostic value (Fig. 11-1). Graham and Johnson[12] recently have reported the presence of various immunoglobulins, complement, and fibrinogen in nerve biopsy specimens from 6 of 16 patients with diabetes. These authors interpreted the presence of these proteins as a manifestation of abnormal basement membrane permeability. In contrast to the polyneuropathies, the mononeuropathies are generally thought to be the result of vascular insufficiency as the result of either vascular occlusion or compression. Although this interpretation is widely accepted, very few morphologic studies have actually demonstrated the vascular lesions in cranial or other peripheral nerves.[13,14]

UREMIC NEUROPATHY

With the longer survival of patients with chronic renal diseases, peripheral neuropathies became recognized as important complications of chronic uremia.[15] The neuropathies are predominantly sensory in nature and may be accompanied by severe dysesthesias of the feet. Muscular weakness and wasting is less common. The severity of the neuropathies correlated poorly with the degree of uremia. Although the biochemical basis is unclear, the neuropathy can be controlled partially by dialysis and even more completely by renal transplantation.

Pathologic studies have shown distal axonal degeneration accompanied by secondary demyelination.[16,17]Although these morphologic studies contributed greatly to our understanding of the concept of segmental demyelination sec-

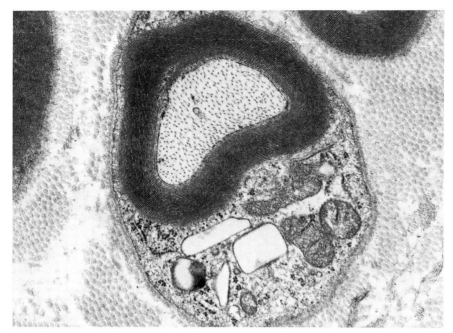

Figure 11–1. Electron micrograph of an intramuscular nerve twig within a muscle biopsy specimen from a patient with diabetic neuropathy. Note the relatively thick basement membrane around the Schwann cell, and the numerous intracytoplasmic lipid inclusions. ×30,000.

ondary to axonal atrophy and degeneration, the histopathologic changes are by themselves not morphologically distinctive.

PORPHYRIC NEUROPATHY

The porphyrias are a group of hereditary disorders resulting in abnormal biosynthesis of porphyrins and porphyrin precursors. Among these disorders, only the so-called hepatic porphyrias are accompanied by neuropathies. The neuropathies are seen most often during acute attacks precipitated by administration of various drugs.[18] The manifestations of the neuropathy include muscular weakness which may begin in the upper extremities. The weakness is often more marked proximally than distally and may be asymmetrical in distribution. Abdominal pain, sensory deficits, and autonomic dysfunction are also common manifestations. The cerebrospinal fluid may show an elevation in protein content, with relatively few cells. Occasionally these cases have been confused with the Guillain–Barré syndrome.[19] Histopathologic studies have shown predominantly axonal degeneration (Figs. 11–2 and 11–3).

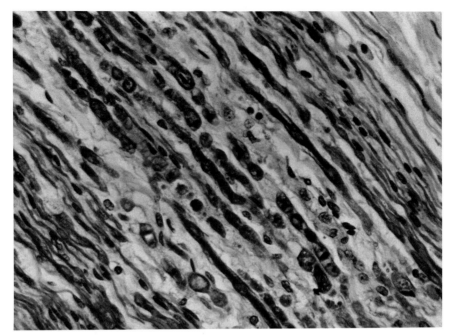

Figure 11-2. Postmortem nerve specimen from a 19-year-old man with acute intermittent porphyria. The patient died 13 days after the onset of an attack that was accompanied by severe peripheral neuropathy. The nerve shows severe axonal degeneration. Trichrome, ×420.

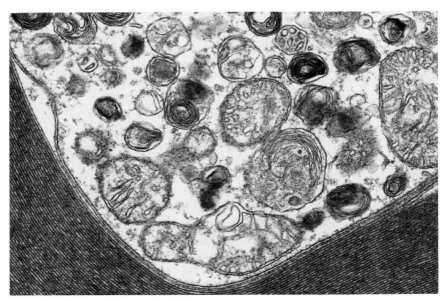

Figure 11-3. Porphyric neuropathy, same patient as in Figure 11-2. Electron micrograph showing the degenerating axoplasmic organelles, including lamellar dense bodies. ×60,000.

NUTRITIONAL NEUROPATHIES

Nutritional deficiencies, especially deficiencies among the group B vitamins, are responsible for an important group of peripheral neuropathies. Some of these neuropathies are due to multiple vitamin deficiencies rather than deficiency of a single vitamin. In the United States, these neuropathies are encountered predominantly in poorly nourished individuals who are also alcoholics. The so-called "alcoholic neuropathy" is attributed primarily to thiamine deficiency[20] although other vitamin deficiencies and the direct neurotoxic effects of alcohol may be contributory factors. The clinical manifestations of alcoholic neuropathy are those of a mixed motor and sensory neuropathy affecting the lower extremities more severely than the upper extremities. In contrast to older reports emphasizing demyelination, more recent pathologic studies have disclosed predominantly axonal degeneration with only secondary segmental demyelination.[21,22] Axonal degeneration was also found to be the predominant pathologic alteration in nerve biopsy specimens from nonalcoholic patients with beriberi neuropathy.[23]

A pyridoxine deficiency neuropathy, manifested predominantly by dysesthesias, may occur in patients receiving isoniazid for treatment of tuberculosis. Pathologic studies have shown axonal degeneration accompanied by degenerative changes in the posterior columns of the spinal cord.[24] Furthermore, it has been suggested that some of the neurologic manifestations attributed to pellagra may actually be due to the effects of pyridoxine deficiency on the central and peripheral nervous systems.[20] Paradoxically, the excessive ingestion of pyridoxine has also been shown to cause a sensory neuropathy. Correlative animal studies have disclosed degeneration of ganglion cells.[25]

Vitamin B_{12} deficiency, secondary to inadequate intrinsic factor production by the stomach or secondary to intestinal malabsorption, is a well-recognized cause of neurologic disease. Most authors attribute the clinical manifestations to a myelopathy, subacute combined degeneration of the spinal cord. However, Pallis and Lewis[26] regard peripheral neuropathy as the most common neurologic manifestation of vitamin B_{12} deficiency. Morphologic studies of peripheral nerve specimens from patients with vitamin B_{12} deficiency states have been less extensive than in some of the other vitamin deficiencies. The often-quoted study by Greenfield and Carmichael[27] emphasized a reduction in the number of large myelin sheaths. A somewhat more recent study by Bischoff et al.[28] indicated axonal involvement. We have encountered a giant axonal neuropathy (Figs. 11–4 through 11–6) in a patient who had vitamin B_{12} malabsorption.[29]

Vitamin E deficiency has been studied extensively in various laboratory animals and is known to produce neurologic abnormalities. In rats, for example, this vitamin deficiency produces a slowly evolving ataxia, and hind limb paralysis. The most conspicuous neuropathologic alterations consisted of demyelination of the posterior columns of the spinal cord, and enlarged, so-called dystrophic axons in the medulla. However, the significance of vitamin E deficiency in human neurologic disease remained more controversial. Recently,

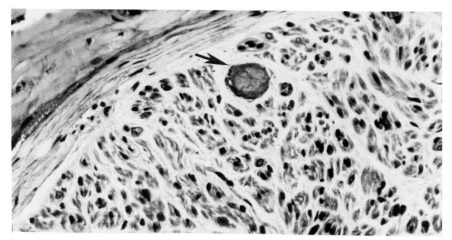

Figure 11-4. Giant axonal enlargement *(arrow)* in a sural nerve biopsy specimen from a 49-year-old man with progressive distal weakness and numbness. The patient was found to have vitamin B$_{12}$ deficiency secondary to intestinal malabsorption. Trichrome, ×420.

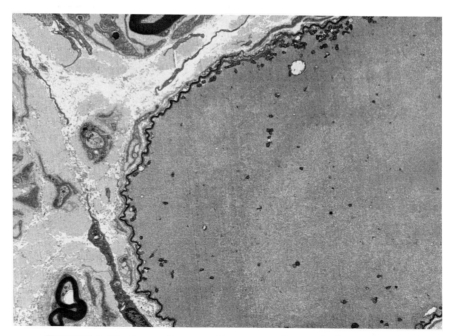

Figure 11-5. Giant axonal neuropathy, same patient as in Figure 11-4. This electron micrograph shows the axonal enlargement to be filled with neurofilaments and surrounded by a thin myelin sheath. ×4000.

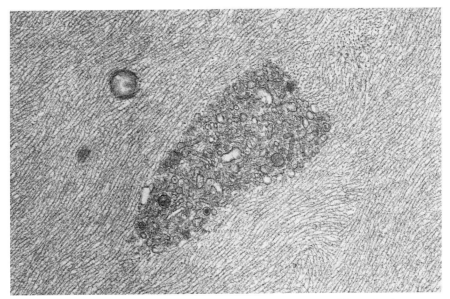

Figure 11-6. Giant axonal neuropathy, same patient as in Figure 11-4. Higher-magnification electron micrograph showing the neurofilaments surrounding small areas containing other organelles. × 42,500.

reports have appeared suggesting that prolonged deficiency of this vitamin also adversely affects the human nervous system. Sung et al.[30] have found large numbers of dystrophic axons in the gracile nuclei of children and young adults with biliary atresia or cystic fibrosis (Fig. 11-7). Furthermore, the dystrophic axons were more numerous in those patients who had not received supplemental vitamin E. Rosenblum et al.[31] described a progressive neurologic syndrome in children with chronic cholestatic liver disease and low serum vitamin E levels. Neuropathologic studies disclosed the presence of dystrophic axons, demyelination of the posterior columns of the spinal cord, and loss of large myelinated fibers from peripheral nerves. Myelin disruption and degenerative changes at the Schmidt–Lantermann incisures also have been described in sural nerve specimens from children with cholestatic liver disease.[32] Dystrophic axons, axonal degeneration of peripheral nerves, and lipid accumulation in Schwann cells have been described in adults with vitamin E deficiency following small bowel resection[33] or acquired intestinal malabsorption.[34]

Sensory neuropathies, presumably nutritional in nature, have been reported as complications of gastric partitioning for morbid obesity[35] and in association with parenteral hyperalimentation.[36] Postmortem studies on a patient with gastric partitioning disclosed severe demyelination of proximal peripheral nerves and vacuolization of anterior horn motor neurons. The vacuoles were thought to result from abnormal accumulations of lipids.

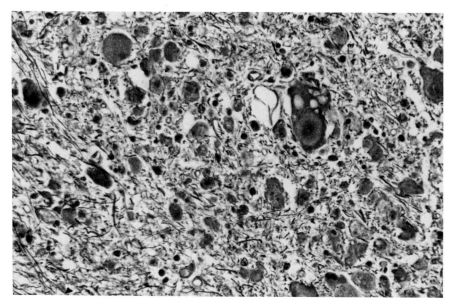

Figure 11-7. Dystrophic axons in the gracile nucleus of an adult with cystic fibrosis. Bodian, ×410.

TOXIC NEUROPATHIES

Under certain circumstances, a wide variety of chemical compounds may produce peripheral neuropathies. These compounds range from common therapeutic agents to exotic environmental contaminants. In most patients, the evolution of the neuropathy is subacute or chronic, reflecting recurrent or persistent exposure. Despite their diverse composition and possibly varied sites of intracellular injury, the majority of these neurotoxic compounds produce mixed motor and sensory neuropathies. Generally the manifestations are symmetrical and affect the lower extremities more severely than the upper extremities. However, there are some noteworthy exceptions, such as the predominance of sensory involvement in the peripheral neuropathies due to arsenic and cisplatin and the asymmetrical, predominantly motor involvement in the peripheral neuropathy due to lead intoxication. Some of the toxic agents simultaneously affect the central nervous system. Depending upon the agent, this can be manifested by encephalopathy, cerebellar dysfunction, or myelopathy with dorsal column dysfunction.

In most of the toxic neuropathies, the pathogenesis appears to be distal axonal degeneration.[37-39] This is often accompanied by varying degrees of secondary demyelination. Unfortunately, the morphologic changes produced by many of these diverse compounds are nearly indistinguishable from one another (Figs. 11-8 through 11-10). For this reason, nerve biopsy is rarely in-

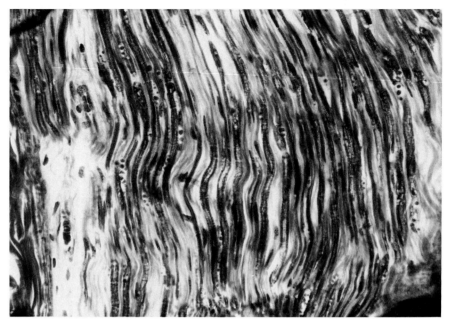

Figure 11-8. Sural nerve biopsy specimen from a 51-year-old man with vincristine neuropathy. Note the numerous fibers undergoing axonal degeneration. Similar alterations can be seen in many other toxic neuropathies. Trichrome, ×500.

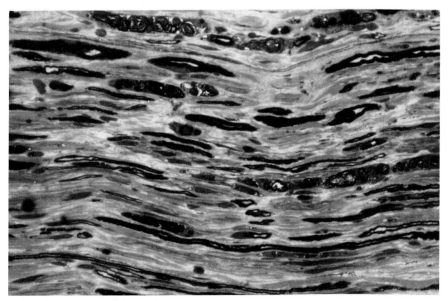

Figure 11-9. Epoxy-embedded section of a sural nerve biopsy specimen from a 39-year-old man with arsenical neuropathy. Note the scattered fibers undergoing axonal degeneration. Toluidine blue, ×500.

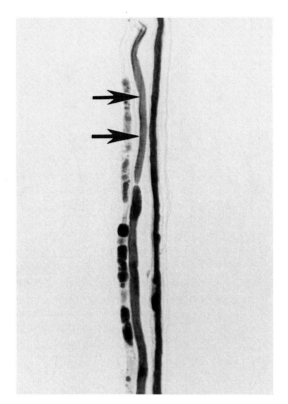

Figure 11-10. Teased nerve fiber preparation from a sural nerve biopsy specimen from a 43-year-old woman with peripheral neuropathy and myopathy, secondary to injudicious self-medication with colchicine. Note the presence of myelin ovoids, indicating axonal degeneration, and an adjacent fiber with a thinly myelinated internode *(arrows)*. ×190.

dicated in the routine diagnostic evaluation of patients suspected of having toxic neuropathies. Even extensive examination of peripheral nerve specimens at the time of autopsy will rarely disclose the cause of the neuropathy, although the pattern of involvement can be studied in detail.

The histopathologic alterations associated with these peripheral neuropathies are often best demonstrated in teased fiber preparations. Among the individual teased fibers, those undergoing axonal degeneration appear as rows of myelin ovoids. In paraffin-embedded sections, the axonal degeneration is less conspicuous and is seen in the form of scattered digestion chambers. These appear as dark-stained fragments of axonal debris contained within small vacuoles. Schwann cell proliferation follows the axonal degeneration, and when the course of the neuropathy is protracted the affected nerves may appear to contain an increased number of endoneurial nuclei. Eventually, endoneurial fibrosis ensues. Nerve fiber regeneration often occurs concurrently with the degeneration and is manifested by small groups or clusters of tiny neurites surrounded by a common basement membrane. These axonal clusters are best seen by light microscopy in epoxy-embedded sections or by electron microscopy.

Morphologically distinctive features may be encountered in a few of the toxic neuropathies. Peripheral nerve specimens from at least some of the patients with peripheral neuropathies due to exposure to n-hexane and methyl butyl ketone have shown giant axonal enlargements.[35] These are focal axonal swellings that are encountered along the course of peripheral nerves proximal to the nodes of Ranvier. The axonal enlargements are filled with neurofilaments. They presumably result from local impairment of axonal transport mediated by 2,5-hexanedione, a highly neurotoxic catabolite of both n-hexane and methyl butyl ketone. The myelin sheaths covering the giant axonal enlargements are thinned and partially retracted. The secondary myelin alterations may be responsible for the slowed nerve conduction velocities that are characteristically encountered in patients with these disorders. Morphologically similar axonal enlargements may be seen in the dorsal columns of the spinal cord.

References

1. Thomas PK, Eliasson SG: Diabetic neuropathy. In Dyck PJ, Thomas PK, Lambert EH, Bunge R (eds): Peripheral Neuropathy. Philadelphia, Saunders, 1984, Vol 2, pp 1773–1810.
2. Powell HC: Pathology of diabetic neuropathy: New observations, new hypotheses. Lab Invest 49:515–518, 1983.
3. Brown MJ, Asbury AK: Diabetic neuropathy. Ann Neurol 15:2–12, 1984.
4. Brown MJ, Martin JR, Asbury AK: Painful diabetic neuropathy. A morphometric study. Arch Neurol 33:164–171, 1976.
5. Calverly JR, Mulder DW: Femoral neuropathy. Neurology 10:963–967, 1960.
6. Ballin RHM, Thomas PK: Hypertrophic changes in diabetic neuropathy. Acta Neuropathol 11:93–102, 1968.
7. Behse F, Buchthal F, Carlsen F: Nerve biopsy and conduction studies in diabetic neuropathy. J Neurol Neurosurg Psychiatry 40:1072–1082, 1977.
8. Dyck PJ, Sherman WR, Hallcher LM, et al.: Human diabetic endoneurial sorbitol, fructose, and myo-inositol related to sural nerve morphometry. Ann Neurol 8:590–596, 1980.
9. Sugimura K, Dyck PJ: Sural nerve myelin thickness and axis cylinder caliber in human diabetes. Neurology 31:1087–1091, 1981.
10. Johnson PC, Brendel K, Meezan E: Human diabetic perineurial cell basement membrane thickening. Lab Invest 44:265–270, 1981.
11. Johnson PC: Thickening of the human dorsal root ganglion perineurial cell basement membrane in diabetes mellitus. Muscle Nerve 6:561–565, 1983.
12. Graham AR, Johnson PC: Direct immunofluorescence findings in peripheral nerve from patients with diabetic neuropathy. Ann Neurol 17:450–454, 1985.
13. Asbury AK, Aldredge H, Hershberg R, Fisher CM: Oculomotor palsy in diabetes mellitus: A clinico-pathological study. Brain 93:555–566, 1970.
14. Raff MC, Asbury AK: Ischemic mononeuropathy and mononeuropathy multiplex in diabetes mellitus. N Engl J Med 279:17–22, 1968.

15. Asbury AK: Uremic neuropathy. In Dyck PJ, Thomas PK, Lambert EH, Bunge R (eds): Peripheral Neuropathy. Philadelphia, Saunders, 1984, Vol 2, pp 1811–1825.

16. Said G, Boudier L, Selva J, et al.: Different patterns of uremic polyneuropathy: Clinicopathologic study. Neurology 33:567–574, 1983.

17. Dyck PJ, Johnson WJ, Lambert EH, O'Brien PC: Segmental demyelination secondary to axonal degeneration in uremic neuropathy. Mayo Clin Proc 46:400–431, 1971.

18. Ridley A: Porphyric neuropathy. In Dyck PJ, Thomas PK, Lambert EH, Bunge R (eds): Peripheral Neuropathy. Philadelphia, Saunders, 1984, Vol 2, pp 1704–1716.

19. Feit H, Tindall RSA, Glasberg M: Sources of error in the diagnosis of Guillain–Barré syndrome. Muscle Nerve 5:111–117, 1982.

20. Victor M: Polyneuropathy due to nutritional deficiency and alcoholism. In Dyck PJ, Thomas PK, Lambert EH, Bunge R (eds): Peripheral Neuropathy. Philadelphia, Saunders, 1984, Vol 2, pp 1899–1940.

21. Walsh JC, McLeod JG: Alcoholic neuropathy: An electrophysiological and histological study. J Neurol Sci 10:457–469, 1970.

22. Behse F, Buchthal F: Alcoholic neuropathy: Clinical, electrophysiological and biopsy findings. Ann Neurol 2:95–110, 1977.

23. Ohnishi A, Tsuji S, Igisu H, et al.: Beriberi neuropathy. Morphometric study of sural nerve. J Neurol Sci 45:177–190, 1980.

24. Blakemore WF: Isoniazid. In Spencer PS, Schaumburg HH (eds): Experimental and Clinical Neurotoxicology. Baltimore, Williams & Wilkins, 1980, pp 476–489.

25. Schaumburg H, Kaplan J, Windebank A, et al.: Sensory neuropathy from pyridoxine abuse. N Engl J Med 309:445–448, 1983.

26. Pallis CA, Lewis PD: The Neurology of Gastrointestinal Disease. London, Saunders, 1974, pp 30–97.

27. Greenfield JG, Carmichael EA: The peripheral nerves in cases of subacute combined degeneration of the cord. Brain 58:483–491, 1935.

28. Bischoff A, Lutschg J, Meier C: Polyneuropathie bei Vitamin-B12-und Folsauereremangel. Klinisch-histopathologische Studie mit elektronmikroskopischer Analyse des Nervus suralis. Munch Med Wochenschr 117:1593–1598, 1975.

29. Schochet SS Jr, Chesson AL Jr: Giant axonal neuropathy: Possibly secondary to vitamin B$_{12}$ malabsorption. Acta Neuropathol 40:79–83, 1977.

30. Sung JH, Park SH, Mastri AR, Warwick WJ: Axonal dystrophy in the gracile nucleus in congenital biliary atresia and cystic fibrosis (mucoviscidosis): Beneficial effect of vitamin E therapy. J Neuropathol Exp Neurol 39:584–597, 1980.

31. Rosenblum JL, Keating JP, Prensky AL, Nelson JS: A progressive neurologic syndrome in children with chronic liver disease. N Engl J Med 304:503–508, 1981.

32. Werlin SL, Harb JM, Swick H, Blank E: Neuromuscular dysfunction and ultrastructural pathology in children with chronic cholestasis and vitamin E deficiency. Ann Neurol 13:291–296, 1983.

33. Bertoni JM, Abraham FA, Fall HF, Itabashi HH: Small bowel resection with vitamin E deficiency and progressive cerebellar syndrome. Neurology 34:1046–1052, 1984.

34. Weder B, Meienberg O, Wildi E, Meier C: Neurologic disorder of vitamin E deficiency in acquired intestinal malabsorption. Neurology 34:1561–1565, 1984.

35. Feit H, Glasberg M, Ireton C, et al.: Peripheral neuropathy and starvation after gastric partitioning for morbid obesity. Ann Intern Med 96:453–455, 1982.

36. May WE: Nutritional sensory neuropathy: An emerging new syndrome. Arch Neurol 41:559–560, 1984.

37. Schaumberg HH, Spencer PS: Human toxic neuropathy due to industrial agents. In

Dyck PJ, Thomas PK, Lambert EH, Bunge R (eds): Peripheral Neuropathy. Philadelphia, Saunders, 1984, Vol 2, pp 2115–2132.

38. Windebank AJ, McCall JT, Dyck PJ: Metal neuropathy. In Dyck PJ, Thomas PK, Lambert EH, Bunge R (eds): Peripheral Neuropathy. Philadelphia, Saunders, 1984, Vol 2, pp 2133–2161.

39. Le Quesne PM, Neuropathy due to drugs. In Dyck PJ, Thomas PK, Lambert EH, Bunge R (eds): Peripheral Neuropathy. Philadelphia, Saunders, 1984, Vol 2, pp 2162–2179.

chapter 12

Hereditary Neuropathies

The hereditary neuropathies are a large, heterogeneous group of diseases. Some are frequently encountered clinically while others are relatively rare. The biochemical basis for some of the more common hereditary neuropathies, such as Charcot–Marie–Tooth disease, remains unknown. Some of the rarer neuropathies are caused by metabolic diseases that affect the peripheral nervous system along with other organ systems. In the case of the latter diseases, the biochemical basis is at least partially known. From the standpoint of diagnosis, morphologic studies often are of greater value in the evaluation of the rarer metabolic neuropathies. In these cases, the morphologic findings may suggest diagnostic categories that can be confirmed biochemically. Unfortunately, the morphologic changes encountered in some of the more common hereditary peripheral neuropathies are less specific.

HYPERTROPHIC CHARCOT–MARIE–TOOTH DISEASE

This disorder is also designated as hereditary motor and sensory neuropathy (HMSN) type I according to the classification utilized by Dyck et al.[1] This is a relatively common disorder which is inherited as an autosomal-dominant trait. The manifestations of the disease show a wide range of severity, reflecting the highly variable expression of this autosomal-dominant gene. Typically, affected individuals develop weakness and atrophy of muscles in the distal portions of their legs during childhood or early adult life. The weakness often results in impaired gait. The atrophy may become quite severe and, in some patients, the lower limbs develop a characteristic "inverted champagne bottle" appearance. The feet frequently have abnormally high arches. Weakness and wasting of the hands develop much later, if at all. Sensory abnormalities are generally not prominent although reflexes are characteristically depressed. About one fourth of the affected patients have palpably enlarged peripheral nerves. Electrodiagnostic studies disclose widespread, abnormally slow nerve conduction velocities that are largely independent of the duration or severity of the disease.[2] Many individuals with this disorder are clinically asymptomatic and are detected only as the result of detailed family studies.

Sural nerve biopsy specimens often show an increased transverse fascicular area and a decrease in the proportion of large myelinated nerve fibers. The most striking feature, however, is the presence of numerous onion bulb formations (Figs. 12-1 and 12-2). These are composed of concentric lamellae of Schwann cells and Schwann cell processes separated by collagen. The details of their structure are best seen by electron microscopy (Fig. 12-3). Routine teased nerve fiber preparations show segmental demyelination and thinly myelinated fibers that result from remyelination. Histopathologic studies of the central nervous system of patients with hypertrophic Charcot–Marie–Tooth disease are limited. They have shown mild loss of anterior horn motor neurons and demyelination with gliosis in the dorsal columns of the spinal cord.[3] Prominent onion bulbs may be seen in the spinal roots.

Because of the characteristic clinical features, peripheral nerve biopsies are rarely needed in the routine diagnostic evaluation of these patients. Nevertheless, detailed quantitative morphologic studies by Dyck et al.[1] have contributed enormously to a better understanding of this disease. Although demyelination and remyelination along with onion bulb formations are the most obvious alterations, these authors' studies have suggested that the myelin changes are

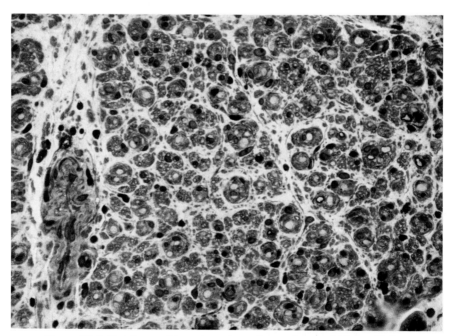

Figure 12-1. Sural nerve biopsy specimen from a 9-year-old boy with hypertrophic Charcot-Marie-Tooth disease. Numerous onion bulbs are evident in this plastic-embedded section. Polychrome stain, ×500.

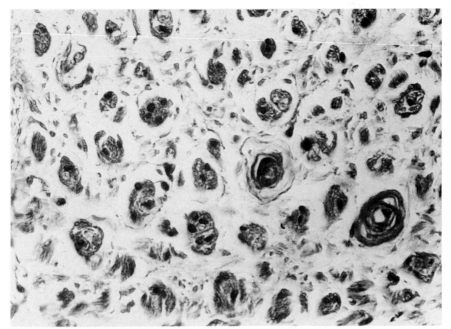

Figure 12-2. Sural nerve biopsy specimen from a 40-year-old man with hypertrophic Charcot–Marie–Tooth disease. The patient had difficulty walking and running since childhood. He had peroneal atrophy and high arches. Other members of his family were similarly affected. PAS–hematoxylin, ×800.

secondary to axonal atrophy. There is some evidence indicating that this may be the result of impaired axonal transport.[4] Recently, some cases of hypertrophic Charcot–Marie–Tooth disease have been shown to be associated with the Duffy blood group.[5] Thus it would appear that this clinical disorder is actually a group of at least two different diseases.

NEURONAL CHARCOT–MARIE–TOOTH DISEASE

This disorder is also designated as HMSN type II according to the classification utilized by Dyck et al.[1] Although the disease is also inherited as an autosomal-dominant trait, it is generally regarded as a separate disorder, distinct from the more common hypertrophic Charcot–Marie–Tooth disease. The two conditions are most clearly distinguished electrophysiologically. In hypertrophic Charcot–Marie–Tooth disease, nerve conduction velocities are diffusely and severely reduced, while in neuronal Charcot–Marie–Tooth disease the nerve conduction velocities are normal or only mildly reduced.[1,6] In addition, there are at least some differences in their clinical presentations. The

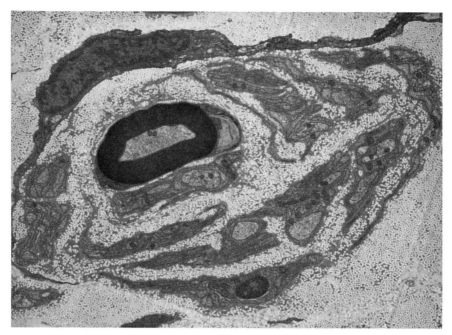

Figure 12-3. Electron micrograph of an onion bulb formation, same patient as in Figure 12-2. ×9000.

patients with the neuronal form of Charcot–Marie–Tooth disease generally have a later onset of clinical manifestations, during or after the second decade. They usually have less severe involvement of the hand muscles, while involvement of the lower limbs may be more severe than in many of the cases of hypertrophic Charcot–Marie–Tooth disease. Furthermore, the peripheral nerves are less likely to be palpably enlarged.

The histopathologic studies of this disease are less comprehensive than those on the hypertrophic form of the disease.[1,7] Nerve specimens from patients with the neuronal form of Charcot–Marie–Tooth disease generally show reduction in the number of large myelinated fibers (Fig. 12-4). However, the transverse fascicular area is nearly normal and there are few, if any, onion bulb formations (Fig. 12-5). The peripheral nerve changes have been regarded to be the result of axonal atrophy that preferentially affects the neurons innervating the lower limbs.[1] Detailed autopsy studies have not yet been reported.

DEJERINE-SOTTAS DISEASE

Dejerine–Sottas disease is a relatively rare, severe form of hypertrophic neuropathy. This disease is designated as HMSN type III according to the classification utilized by Dyck et al.[1] In contrast to the more common Charcot-

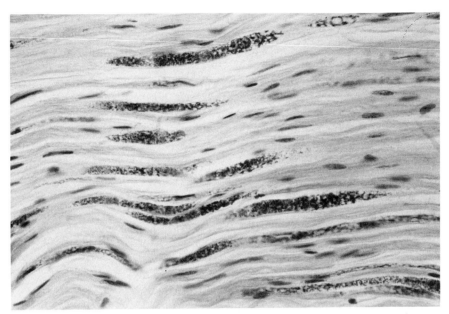

Figure 12-4. Sural nerve biopsy from a 33-year-old woman with neuronal Charcot–Marie–Tooth disease. The biopsy shows a marked loss of myelinated nerve fibers but no onion bulb formations. Trichrome, ×550.

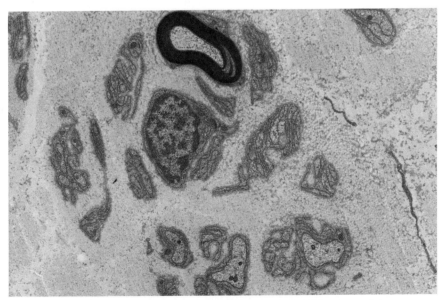

Figure 12-5. Electron micrograph showing stacks of Schwann cell processes (bands of Büngner) resulting from axonal degeneration but no onion bulbs. Same patient as in Figure 12-4. ×9000.

Marie–Tooth disease, this disorder is inherited as an autosomal-recessive trait. The manifestations of the disease appear in infancy, with delayed motor development and weakness. The weakness becomes generalized although it may be manifest initially in the lower limbs. Walking is often severely impaired by the time the patient reaches childhood. The motor impairments are accompanied by distal sensory deficits affecting touch, position, and vibration more than pain and temperature. The affected children are often short and have severe skeletal abnormalities including kyphoscoliosis and deformities of the feet and hands. The peripheral nerves are often palpably enlarged. Electrophysiologic studies consistently demonstrate markedly reduced nerve conduction velocities. The cerebrospinal fluid commonly contains increased protein.

Histopathologic studies disclose enlarged peripheral nerves with an increased transverse fascicular area. The nerves show a marked reduction in the number of myelinated fibers (Fig. 12–6). Those remaining tend to be relatively small. Teased fiber preparations disclose long segments of nerve fibers that are devoid of myelin. However, the most striking morphologic feature is the presence of large numbers of unusually prominent onion bulb formations (Fig. 12–7). In epoxy sections and by electron microscopy, these often appear quite complex, with numerous Schwann cell processes participating in their formation

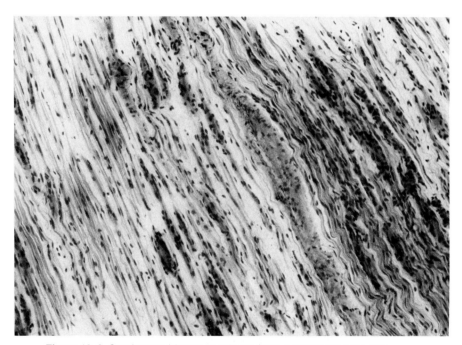

Figure 12-6. Sural nerve biopsy specimen from a 7-year-old boy with Dejerine–Sottas disease. Note the reduction in the number of myelinated nerve fibers and the increased mucoid material in the endoneurium. H&E, ×175.

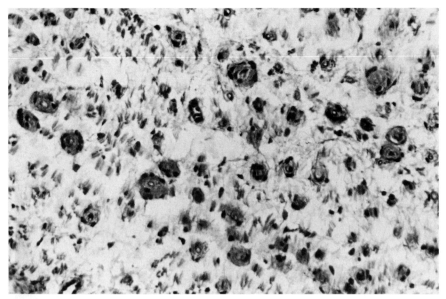

Figure 12-7. Dejerine–Sottas disease, same patient as in Figure 12-6. Note the prominent but widely seperated onion bulbs. H&E, ×400.

(Fig. 12–8). The pathogenesis of this disorder remains unknown. Axonal atrophy with secondary demyelination has been suggested by Dyck et al.[1]

HEREDITARY SENSORY NEUROPATHIES

There are several hereditary neuropathies that are characterized predominantly by sensory deficits along with varying degrees of autonomic dysfunction.[8] All are quite rare. The individual diseases have been delineated and classified according to the patterns of inheritance, age of onset, severity, and presence of secondary features such as plantar ulcers and acral mutilation.

The dominantly inherited sensory neuropathy, otherwise known as hereditary sensory and autonomic neuropathy, type I,[8] generally becomes manifest during late childhood or early adult life. The lower extremities are affected more severely than the upper extremities. The sensory deficits are predominantly loss of pain and temperature perception. As a result, the affected individuals sustain multiple painless foot injuries and may develop secondary infections. These eventually lead to plantar ulcers and foot deformities. Histopathologic studies of peripheral nerve biopsy specimens disclose severe loss of unmyelinated nerve fibers and mild to moderate loss of myelinated fibers.

The autosomal-recessive hereditary sensory neuropathy, otherwise known as hereditary sensory and autonomic neuropathy, type II,[8] generally becomes manifest earlier in life, even in infancy. Both the upper and lower extremities

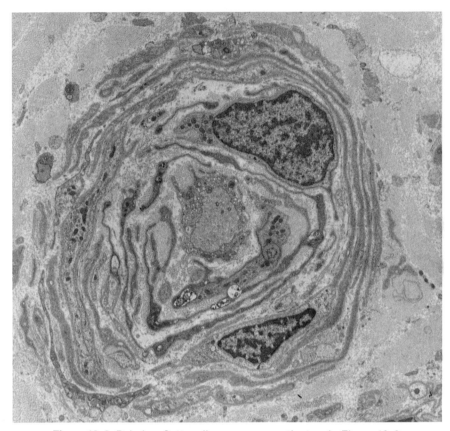

Figure 12-8. Dejerine–Sottas disease, same patient as in Figure 12–6. This electron micrograph shows one of the large, complex onion bulb formations. ×6000.

are affected. As a result, the affected individuals sustain multiple traumatic injuries of the hands as well as the feet. In this disorder, the histopathologic findings are the converse of those encountered in the dominantly inherited disease. Peripheral nerve biopsy specimens have shown severe loss of myelinated fibers with milder involvement of the unmyelinated fibers.[9] In addition, some of the patients have shown prominent vacuolation of endoneurial fibroblasts.[10] However, this morphologic feature is not unique to this disorder.[11]

Familial dysautonomia or the Riley–Day syndrome has been classified among these disorders and designated as hereditary sensory and autonomic neuropathy, type III.[8] This autosomal-recessive disorder is found predominantly among Ashkanazi Jews. It is characterized by prominent autonomic dysfunction along with milder sensory deficits. The affected individuals typically have smooth tongues lacking fungiform papillae. Peripheral nerve biopsy specimens show predominantly a loss of unmyelinated fibers. In addition, autopsy studies have shown numerous abnormalities of the central nervous system.[12]

Although the spinocerebellar degenerations affect the central nervous system more severely than the peripheral nervous system, peripheral nerves from these patients may display demyelination secondary to axonal degeneration.[8,13] Generally, the changes are more severe among the larger myelinated fibers. Although the metabolic basis for these diseases remains unsettled, a deficiency of mitochondrial malic enzyme activity has been demonstrated in fibroblasts from patients with Friedreich's ataxia.[14]

CHILDHOOD GIANT AXONAL NEUROPATHY

Childhood giant axonal neuropathy is a rare, progressive neuropathy of childhood. The disorder was originally described by Berg et al.[15] and Asbury et al.[16] This patient, along with those described subsequently, have displayed rather characteristic clinical features. The onset of symptoms is generally before the age of 3 years. In addition to the manifestations of a mixed motor and sensory neuropathy, the patients generally display evidence of central nervous system involvement. Most often this is in the form of ataxia and nystagmus. Several of the patients have also had impaired speech and mild mental retardation. Most but not all of the children have unusually kinky hair. In addition, the hair may be abnormally light-colored. The occurrence of more than one case in a few families has suggested an autosomal-recessive inheritance pattern.[17-19]

Peripheral nerve specimens from these patients have shown highly characteristic morphologic features. There are multiple focal enlargements filled with neurofilaments (Figs. 12–9 and 12–10). These are often adjacent to the nodes of Ranvier. These axonal enlargements are similar to the ones seen in association with hexacarbon intoxication although they generally contain more osmiophilic granular material. In addition, abnormal aggregations of filaments may be seen in other types of cells, such as Schwann cells (Fig. 12–11), fibroblasts, and endothelial cells.[19,20] This feature has been interpreted as morphologic evidence of a systemic disorder of cytoplasmic microfilaments. Recent biochemical studies have suggested that the filaments have a normal composition and that the genetic defect involves the organization of the intermediate filaments.[21]

TOMACULOUS NEUROPATHY

The term "tomaculous neuropathy" has been used to describe certain neuropathies that are characterized morphologically by the presence of multifocal-enlargements along the course of peripheral nerve fibers. The enlargements

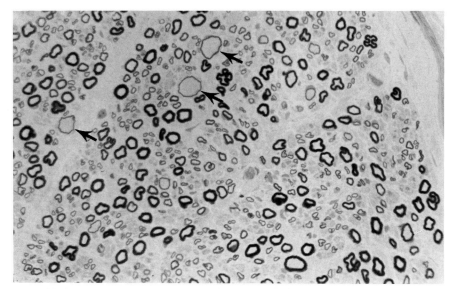

Figure 12-9. Epoxy-embedded section of a sural nerve biopsy specimen from an 8-year-old boy with giant axonal neuropathy. Note the axonal enlargements *(arrows)* surrounded by thinned myelin sheaths. Paraphenylenediamine, × 420. *(Specimen courtesy of Dr. Peter W. Lampert.)*

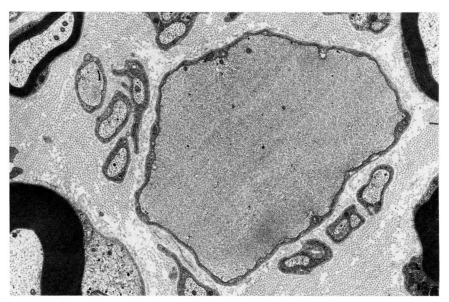

Figure 12-10. Electron micrograph showing one of the axonal enlargements filled with neurofilaments. ×9000. *(Specimen courtesy of Dr. Peter W. Lampert.)*

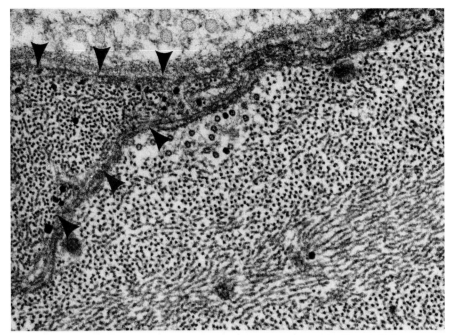

Figure 12-11. Giant axonal neuropathy, same patient as in Figure 12-9. The abnormal accumulation of filaments occurs in both the axon and associated Schwann cell cytoplasm *(indicated by arrowheads).* ×90,000. *(Specimen courtesy of Dr. Peter W. Lampert.)*

are fusiform or sausage-shaped, hence the term "tomaculous" neuropathy. Tomacula have been described in sural nerve biopsy specimens from patients with hereditary pressure-sensitive neuropathies[22,23] and in rare patients with familial brachial plexopathies.[23,24] The patients with the pressure-sensitive neuropathies have recurrent motor and sensory neuropathies that are precipitated by relatively minor trauma. These neuropathies are generally painless. By contrast, the familial brachial plexus neuropathies are often preceded by pain and may be precipitated by infection or immunization.

In contrast to the giant axonal neuropathies, the tomacula result from abnormalities of the myelin sheath and consist of abnormally thick or redundant loops of myelin. They are encountered most often in a paranodal location. The enlargements measure 30 to 40 μm in diameter and up to 250 μm in length. As many as one third of the fibers in a teased fiber preparation may harbor tomacula. In addition, the affected nerves often show demyelination and remyelination (Fig. 12-12). The diagnosis of tomaculous neuropathy must be made with caution since preparation artifacts, especially in epoxy sections and electron micrographs, can closely mimic the appearance of tomacula.

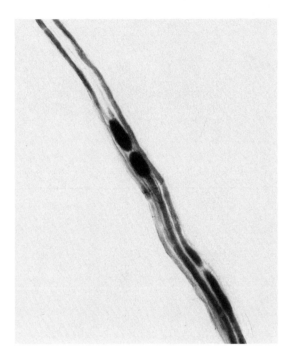

Figure 12-12. Teased fiber preparation from a sural nerve biopsy specimen from a 28-year-old man with pressure-sensitive tomaculous neuropathy. Note the focal enlargements along thinly myelinated nerve fibers. Electron microscopy showed the enlargements to be composed of redundant myelin lamellae. ×175.

KRABBE'S DISEASE

Krabbe's disease, or globoid cell leukodystrophy, is a rare autosomal-recessive disorder due to a deficiency of galactocerebroside beta-galactosidase deficiency.[25] Since galactocerebroside is a constituent of the myelin sheath, the brain and peripheral nerves are the organs that are predominantly affected. The clinical manifestations of the disease usually become apparent between the ages of 3 and 6 months and include excessive irritability, rapid mental and motor deterioration, and eventually blindness and decerebration. Death generally ensues by the age of 2 years although a few cases with later onset of symptoms and longer survival have been recorded.

Grossly, the brains are small with a reduction in the volume of the white matter and a corresponding dilatation of the ventricular system. The remaining white matter is abnormally firm, discolored, and often focally cavitated. The small cavities are most evident in the corpus callosum, internal capsules, and pyramidal tracts. Histologic examination reveals little stainable myelin and a reduction in the number of oligodendrocytes. However, the most characteristic feature is the presence of globoid cells (Fig. 12-13). These are large, uni- or multinucleated macrophages with abundant PAS-positive cytoplasm. They are often aggregated about blood vessels. The formation of the globoid cells is a

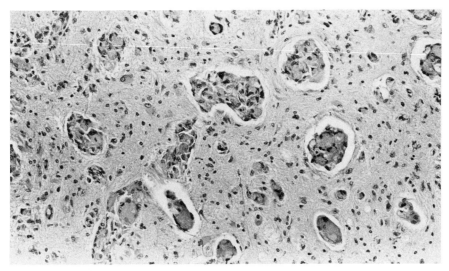

Figure 12–13. Krabbe's disease; brain tissue from a 10-month-old girl showing typical globoid cells. H&E, ×210.

morphologically distinctive response to the presence of uncatabolized intracytoplasmic galactocerebroside. By electron microscopy, the deposits of cerebroside usually appear as elongated, multiangular profiles. Occasionally, longitudinally striated, twisted tubules are also seen. The reduction in the number of oligodendrocytes and deficiency in myelin is attributed to the presence of small but significant amounts of psychosine. This is a highly toxic compound that also accumulates because of the deficiency of galactocerebroside beta-galactosidase.[26]

Involvement of the peripheral nerves, although regularly present, tends to be overshadowed by the central nervous system manifestations. Deep tendon reflexes may be depressed or absent, and nerve conduction velocities are commonly reduced, reflecting demyelination.[27] Peripheral nerve specimens may show a decreased number of large myelinated fibers and segmental demyelination. Foamy histiocytes may be scattered in the endoneurial connective tissue and aggregated about endoneurial blood vessels (Fig. 12–14). These macrophages do not, however, have the characteristic appearance of globoid cells. By electron microscopy, a wide variety of abnormal lipid profiles may be encountered in Schwann cells and macrophages (Fig. 12–15). The deposits within the macrophage more closely resemble the cerebroside deposits found within the globoid cells in the brain.[28] Peripheral nerve involvement is reported to be less prominent in cases of late-onset globoid cell leukodystrophy than in the usual infantile cases of Krabbe's disease.[25]

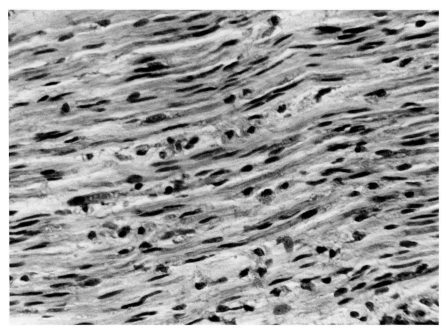

Figure 12-14. Postmortem sural nerve specimen from the same patient as in Figure 12-13. The nerve contains increased numbers of endoneurial and perivascular macrophages, but no true globoid cells as seen in the central nervous system. Trichrome, ×440.

METACHROMATIC LEUKODYSTROPHY

Metachromatic leukodystrophy, otherwise known as sulfatide lipidosis, is due to deficiency of one or more cerebroside sulfatases or a protein necessary for the activity of these enzymes.[29] The more common late-infantile and juvenile forms are thought to be inherited as autosomal-recessive traits. Since sulfatides are constituents of many membranes, a wide variety of tissues in addition to the central and peripheral nervous system are affected in metachromatic leukodystrophy. The disease may become apparent at any time from infancy to adulthood. The clinical manifestations of the late infantile and juvenile forms include arrested development, impaired motor function and speech, blindness, deafness, seizures, and eventually decerebration. Dementia and movement disorders are prominent among the manifestations in adult patients. Patients with the variant associated with multiple sulfatase deficiencies have hepatomegaly and mild skeletal abnormalities, in addition to the usual manifestations of late-infantile metachromatic leukodystrophy.

The cerebral white matter is firm and rubbery and may have an abnormal gray to tan color. Histologically, there is a reduction in stainable myelin and

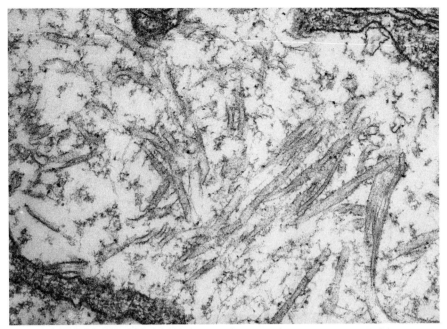

Figure 12–15. Krabbe's disease, same patient as in Figure 12–13. By electron microscopy, the lipid deposits in the endoneurial macrophages appear as prismatic or tubular structures and resemble the cerebroside deposits in the cerebral globoid cells. ×90,000.

a decrease in the number of oligodendrocytes. This is most marked centrally, with relative sparing of the subcortical arcuate fibers. Throughout the white matter, there are abnormal deposits of sulfatides, mainly within macrophages. These deposits are metachromatic, PAS-positive, and display a distinctive brown color with the Hirsch–Peiffer reaction. In specimens from patients with multiple sulfatase deficiencies, neurons also contain abnormal deposits of sulfatides. Ultrastructurally, the sulfatide deposits display a variety of configurations. the most characteristic are in the form of stacks of prismatic lamellae and so-called "tuff stone" deposits.

Peripheral nerve involvement has long been recognized as a prominent feature in metachromatic leukodystrophy. This may be evident both clinically and electrophysiologically in the form of reduced nerve conduction velocities. Peripheral nerve specimens may display demyelination and accumulation of macrophages containing deposits of sulfatides (Fig. 12–16). These are best identified by electron microscopy (Fig. 12–17) since the so-called pi-granules may impart spurious staining with the Hirsch–Peiffer reaction.[30]

In both Krabbe's disease and metachromatic leukodystrophy, morphologic studies are generally performed only for confirmation of diagnoses that are now readily established by biochemical demonstration of the enzyme deficiencies.

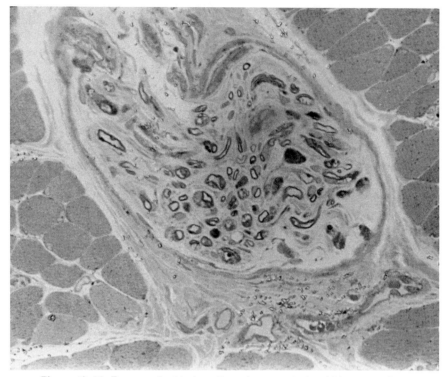

Figure 12-16. Epoxy-embedded section of a nerve twig within a muscle biopsy specimen from a patient with metachromatic leukodystrophy. Note the abnormal deposits of osmiophilic material within Schwann cells. Paraphenylenediamine, ×420.

ADRENOLEUKODYSTROPHY

Adrenoleukodystrophy and related disorders, such as adrenomyeloneuropathy and neonatal adrenoleukodystrophy, are disorders of lipid metabolism that affect predominantly the nervous system and adrenal glands.[31-33] The more common, classical form of adrenoleukodystrophy is inherited as an X-linked disorder and thus occurs predominantly in boys. The clinical manifestations generally appear between the ages of 4 and 8 years and include behavioral changes, intellectual deterioration, visual loss, and progressive motor dysfunction. Seizures have occurred in many of these individuals. The disease usually progresses rapidly, leading to death within a few years. The associated adrenal involvement is highly variable in its expression. Some of the patients have overt adrenal insufficiency that precedes or accompanies the neurologic dysfunction. More often, the adrenal involvement is less pronounced and can only be demonstrated by clinical laboratory studies.

Adrenomyeloneuropathy is less common and affects individuals of both

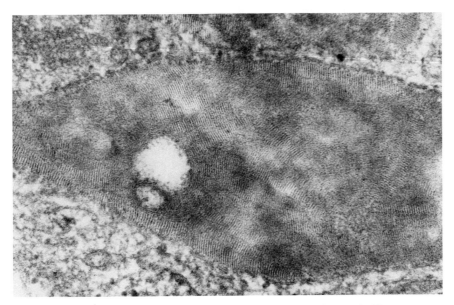

Figure 12-17. Metachromatic leukodystrophy, same patient as in Figure 12-16. This electron micrograph shows the lamellar ultrastructure of the abnormal sulfatide deposits within the Schwann cells. ×140,000.

sexes. The patients often develop adrenal insufficiency in childhood. This is followed by the development of spastic paraparesis and peripheral neuropathy in early adult life. Cerebellar ataxia, intellectual deterioration, and varying degrees of hypogonadism are late manifestations. This form of the disease is more slowly progressive and the patients usually survive to the fourth or fifth decades. Some of the adult and childhood cases show combined features of both the classical disease and adrenomyeloneuropathy.

Neonatal forms of adrenoleukodystrophy have also been described. These forms of the disease are thought to be inherited as autosomal-recessive disorders. The affected infants show severe psychomotor retardation, hypotonia, seizures, and blindness. The adrenal dysfunction is generally inconspicuous. These forms of the disease are rapidly progressive and lead to death at an early age.

Pathologic studies on patients with the classical form of the disease[31] have shown extensive demyelination and focal cavitation of cerebral white matter that is most severe within the posterior temporal, parietal, and occipital lobes. The cerebral lesion may be asymmetrical or bilateral, with involvement of the interhemispheric commissures. The arcuate fibers tend to be spared. Microscopically, the lesions are characterized predominantly by demyelination, loss of oligodendrocytes, and accumulation of lipid-laden macrophages. Reactive astrocytes and perivascular mononuclear cell infiltrates are also seen. Some of the lipid-laden macrophages, especially those near blood vessels, contain PAS-positive material. Ultrastructurally, these cells contain morphologically distinctive, trilaminar, lipid deposits (Fig. 12–18). These are formed by pairs of straight or curved osmiophilic lamellae that are separated by electron-lucent clear spaces. The adrenal cortical cells are enlarged and have striated-appearing cytoplasm. Ultrastructurally, these cells also contain the characteristic trilaminar inclusions.

Pathologic studies on the central nervous system in patients with adrenomyeloneuropathy[32] have shown multiple patchy or confluent areas of demyelination with a less-pronounced loss of oligodendrocytes and fewer lipid-laden macrophages. In addition, reactive astrocytes are less numerous and the perivascular mononuclear cell infiltrates are milder. The spinal cords of these patients show degeneration of the posterior columns, spinocerebellar tracts, and corticospinal tracts. The spinal roots show loss of axons and myelin sheaths. The adrenals show ballooned cortical cells, especially in the zona fasciculata and reticularis. Similar alterations are seen in the testes.

Pathologic studies on tissues from neonatal cases of adrenoleukodystrophy[33] have shown structural abnormalities such as polymicrogyria and heterotopias, in addition to a reduction in the volume of cerebral white matter. Within the white matter were foci of demyelination, gliosis, lipid-laden macrophages, and

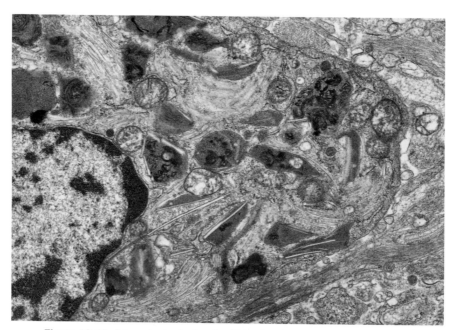

Figure 12–18. Adrenoleukodystrophy. This electron micrograph from a brain biopsy specimen illustrates the appearance of the trilaminar inclusions. In some patients, similar structures have been observed in Schwann cells. ×20,000.

perivascular mononuclear cell infiltrates. The adrenals were small but contained ballooned cortical cells with striated cytoplasm. Abnormal lipid accumulation was also demonstrated in a wide variety of other visceral tissues.

Peripheral nerves have been studied most extensively in patients with adrenomyeloneuropathy. The nerves generally show a reduction in the number of myelinated fibers and endoneurial fibrosis. The characteristic trilaminar lipid inclusions have been observed ultrastructurally within Schwann cells in some of these patients.

Biochemically, the various forms of adrenoleukodystrophy are characterized by abnormal accumulations of very long-chain fatty acids. These compounds are thought to accumulate because of diminished degradation within peroxisomes.[34] The long-chain fatty acids are especially abundant in the cholesterol esters and gangliosides of the brain and adrenals. They also can be demonstrated readily in the blood. Assays of the ratio of C-26 to C-22 fatty acids are currently used as the standard method for definitive diagnosis of these conditions.

References

1. Dyck PJ: Inherited neuronal degeneration and atrophy affecting peripheral motor, sensory, and autonomic neurons. In Dyck PJ, Thomas PK, Lambert EH, Bunge R (eds): Peripheral Neuropathy. Philadelphia, Saunders, 1984, Vol 2, pp 1600–1655.
2. Gutmann L, Fakadej A, Riggs JE: Evolution of nerve conduction abnormalities in children with dominant hypertrophic neuropathy of the Charcot–Marie–Tooth type. Muscle Nerve 6:515–519, 1983.
3. Smith TW, Bhawan J, Kellar RB, DeGirolami U: Charcot–Marie–Tooth disease associated with hypertrophic neuropathy. A neuropathologic study of two cases. J Neuropathol Exp Neurol 39:420–440, 1980.
4. Nukada H, Dyck PJ: Decreased axon caliber and neurofilaments in hereditary motor and sensory neuropathy, type I. Ann Neurol 16:238–241, 1984.
5. Bird TD, Ott J, Giblett ER, et al.: Genetic linkage evidence for heterogeneity in Charcot–Marie–Tooth neuropathy (HMSN type I). Ann Neurol 14:679–684, 1983.
6. Buchthal F, Behse F: Peroneal muscular atrophy (PMA) and related disorders. I. Clinical manifestations as related to biopsy findings, nerve conduction and electromyography. Brain 100:41–66, 1977.
7. Behse F, Buchthal F: Peroneal muscular atrophy (PMA) and related disorders. II. Histological findings in sural nerves. Brain 100:67–85, 1977.
8. Dyck PJ: Neuronal atrophy and degeneration predominantly affecting peripheral sensory and autonomic neurons. In Dyck PJ, Thomas PK, Lambert EH, Bunge R (eds): Peripheral Neuropathy. Philadelphia, Saunders, 1984, Vol 2, pp 1557–1599.
9. Ohta M, Ellefson RD, Lambert EH, Dyck PJ: Hereditary sensory neuropathy, type II. Clinical, electrophysiologic, histologic, and biochemical studies of a Quebec kinship. Arch Neurol 29:23–37, 1973.
10. Schoene WC, Asbury AK, Astrom KE, Masters R: Hereditary sensory neuropathy. A clinical and ultrastructural study. J Neurol Sci 11:463–487, 1970.

11. Asbury AK, Cox SC, Baringer JR: The significance of giant vacuolation of endoneurial fibroblasts. Acta Neuropathol 18:123–131, 1971.

12. Agamanolis DP, Traynor LA: Congenital dysautonomia. A case with a posterior inter-hemispheric cyst and microcephaly. J Neuropathol Exp Neurol 42:469–478, 1983.

13. McCleod JG, Evans WA: Peripheral neuropathy in spinocerebellar degenerations. Muscle Nerve 4:51–61, 1981.

14. Stumpf DA, Parks JK, Eguren LA, Haas R: Friedreich ataxia. III. Mitochondrial malic enzyme deficiency. Neurology 32:221–227, 1982.

15. Berg BO, Rosenberg SH, Asbury AK: Giant axonal neuropathy. Pediatrics 49:894–899, 1972.

16. Asbury AK, Gale MK, Cox SC, et al.: Giant axonal neuropathy — a unique case with segmental neurofilamentous masses. Acta Neuropathol 20:237–247, 1972.

17. Igisu H, Ohta M, Tabira T, et al.: Giant axonal neuropathy. A clinical entity affecting the central as well as the peripheral nervous system. Neurology 25:717–721, 1975.

18. Gambarelli D, Hassoun J, Pellisier JF, et al.: Giant axonal neuropathy. Involvement of peripheral nerve, myenteric plexus and extra-neuronal area. Acta Neuropathol 39:261–269, 1977.

19. Prineas JW, Ouvrier RA, Wright RG, et al.: Giant axonal neuropathy — a generalized disorder of cytoplasmic microfilament formation. J Neuropathol Exp Neurol 35:458–470, 1976.

20. Koch T, Schultz P, Williams R, Lampert P: Giant axonal neuropathy: A childhood disorder of microfilaments. Ann Neurol 1:438–451, 1977.

21. Pena SDJ: Giant axonal neuropathy: An inborn error of organization of intermediate filaments. Muscle Nerve 5:166–172, 1982.

22. Behse F, Buchthal F, Carlsen F, Knappeis GG: Hereditary neuropathy with liability to pressure palsies. Electrophysiological and histopathological aspects. Brain 95:777–794, 1972.

23. Madrid R, Bradley WG: The pathology of neuropathies with focal thickening of the myelin sheath (Tomaculous neuropathy). Studies on the formation of the abnormal myelin sheath. J Neurol Sci 25:415–448, 1975.

24. Bosh EP, Chui HC, Martin MA, Cancilla PA: Brachial plexus involvement in pressure-sensitive neuropathy. Electrophysiological and morphological findings. Ann Neurol 8:620–624, 1980.

25. Suzuki K, Suzuki Y: Galactosylceramide lipidosis: Globoid cell leukodystrophy (Krabbe's disease). In Stanbury JB, Wyngaarden JB, Fredrickson DS, et al. (eds): The Metabolic Basis of Inherited Disease, 5th ed. New York, McGraw-Hill, 1983, pp 857–880.

26. Vanier MT, Svennerholm L: Chemical pathology of Krabbe's disease. III. Ceramide-hexosides and gangliosides of the brain. Acta Paediatr Scand 64:641–648, 1975.

27. Hogan GR, Gutmann L, Chou SM: The peripheral neuropathy of Krabbe's (globoid) leukodystrophy. Neurology 19:1094–1100, 1969.

28. Schochet SS Jr, McCormick WK, Powell GF: Krabbe's disease. A light and electron microscopic study. Acta Neuropathol 36:153–160, 1976.

29. Kolodny EH, Moser HW: Sulfatide lipidosis: Metachromatic leukodystrophy. In Stanbury JB, Wyngaarden JB, Fredrickson DS, et al. (eds): The Metabolic Basis of Inherited Disease, 5th ed. New York, McGraw-Hill, 1983, pp 881–905.

30. Thomas PK, King RHM, Kocen RS, Brett EM: Comparative ultrastructural observations on peripheral nerve abnormalities in the late infantile, juvenile and late onset forms of metachromatic leukodystrophy. Acta Neuropathol 39:237–245, 1977.

31. Schaumburg HH, Powers JM, Raine CS, et al.: Adrenoleukodystrophy. A clinical and pathological study of 17 cases. Arch Neurol 32:577–691, 1975.
32. Schaumburg HH, Powers JM, Raine CS, et al.: Adrenomyeloneuropathy: A probable variant of adrenoleukodystrophy. Neurology 27:1114–1119, 1977.
33. Jaffe R, Crumrine P, Hashida Y, Moser HW: Neonatal adrenoleukodystrophy: Clinical, pathologic, and biochemical delineation of a syndrome affecting both males and females. Am J Pathol 108:100–111, 1982.
34. Moser HW, Moser AE, Singh I, O'Neill BP: Adrenoleukodystrophy: Survey of 303 cases: Biochemistry, diagnosis, and therapy. Ann Neurol 16:628–641, 1984.

Index